ORTHOPEDIC CLINICS OF NORTH AMERICA

www.orthopedic.theclinics.com

New Technologies

January 2019 • Volume 50 • Number 1

ELSEVIER

1600 John F. Kennedy Boulevard • Suite 1800 • Philadelphia, Pennsylvania, 19103-2899.

http://www.orthopedic.theclinics.com

ORTHOPEDIC CLINICS OF NORTH AMERICA Volume 50, Number 1
January 2019 ISSN 0030-5898, ISBN-13: 978-0-323-67536-9

Editor: Lauren Boyle
Developmental Editor: Kristen Helm

Orthopedic Clinics of North America (ISSN 0030-5898) is published quarterly by Elsevier Inc., 360 Park Avenue South, New York, NY 10010-1710. Months of issue are January, April, July, and October. Business and Editorial Offices: 1600 John F. Kennedy Blvd., Suite 1800, Philadelphia, PA 19103-2899. Customer Service Office: 3251 Riverport Lane, Maryland Heights, MO 63043. Periodicals postage paid at New York, NY and additional mailing offices. Subscription prices are $341.00 per year for (US individuals), $749.00 per year for (US institutions), $403.00 per year (Canadian individuals), $914.00 per year (Canadian institutions), $466.00 per year (international individuals), $914.00 per year (international institutions), $100.00 per year (US students), $220.00 per year (Canadian and international students). Foreign air speed delivery is included in all *Clinics* subscription prices. All prices are subject to change without notice. **POSTMASTER:** Send change of address to *Orthopedic Clinics of North America*, **Elsevier Health Sciences Division, Subscription Customer Service, 3251 Riverport Lane, Maryland Heights, MO 63043. Customer Service (orders, claims, online, change of address): Elsevier Health Sciences Division, Subscription Customer Service, 3251 Riverport Lane, Maryland Heights, MO 63043. Tel: 1-800-654-2452 (U.S. and Canada); 314-447-8871 (outside U.S. and Canada). Fax: 314-447-8029. E-mail:** journalscustomerservice-usa@elsevier.com **(for print support);** journalsonlinesupport-usa@elsevier.com **(for online support).**

Reprints. For copies of 100 or more, of articles in this publication, please contact the Commercial Reprints Department, Elsevier Inc., 360 Park Avenue South, New York, NY 10010-1710. Tel.: 212-633-3874; Fax: 212-633-3820; E-mail: reprints@elsevier.com.

Orthopedic Clinics of North America is covered in *MEDLINE/PubMed* (*Index Medicus*), *Cinahl, Excerpta Medica,* and *Cumulative Index to Nursing and Allied Health Literature.*

PROGRAM OBJECTIVE

Orthopedic Clinics of North America offers clinical review articles on the most cutting-edge technologies and techniques in the field, including knee and hip reconstruction, hand and wrist, paediatrics, trauma, shoulder and elbow, and foot and ankle.

TARGET AUDIENCE

Practicing orthopedic surgeons, orthopedic residents, and other healthcare professionals who specialize in orthopedic technologies and techniques for knee and hip reconstruction, hand and wrist, paediatrics, trauma, shoulder and elbow, and foot and ankle.

LEARNING OBJECTIVES

Upon completion of this activity, participants will be able to:
1. Review technologies in pediatric spine surgery
2. Discuss new imaging, diagnostic, and assessment techniques in orthopaedic trauma
3. Recognize emerging technologies in upper extremity surgery

ACCREDITATION

The Elsevier Office of Continuing Medical Education (EOCME) is accredited by the Accreditation Council for Continuing Medical Education (ACCME) to provide continuing medical education for physicians.

The EOCME designates this enduring material for a maximum of 15 *AMA PRA Category 1 Credit*(s)™. Physicians should claim only the credit commensurate with the extent of their participation in the activity.

All other healthcare professionals requesting continuing education credit for this enduring material will be issued a certificate of participation.

DISCLOSURE OF CONFLICTS OF INTEREST

The EOCME assesses conflict of interest with its instructors, faculty, planners, and other individuals who are in a position to control the content of CME activities. All relevant conflicts of interest that are identified are thoroughly vetted by EOCME for fair balance, scientific objectivity, and patient care recommendations. EOCME is committed to providing its learners with CME activities that promote improvements or quality in healthcare and not a specific proprietary business or a commercial interest.

The planning committee, staff, authors and editors listed below have identified no financial relationships or relationships to products or devices they or their spouse/life partner have with commercial interest related to the content of this CME activity:

Yasser Ibrahim Alkhalife, MBBS, SB; Ian Barrett, MD; Michael J. Beebe, MD; Clayton C. Bettin, MD, BS; Lauren Boyle; James H. Calandruccio, MD; Todd K. Conlan, MD; Ameer M. Elbuluk, MD; Ron El-Hawary, MD, MSc, FRCS(C); Reza A. Ghasemi, MD; Matthew Gotlin, MD; James G. Gurney, PhD; Richard Iorio, MD; Alison Kemp; Manesha Lankachandra, MD; Mark Loftin, PhD; Benjamin M. Mauck, MD; Peter N. Mittwede, MD; Anand M. Murthi, MD; David Novikov, BS; Sneha Prabha Narra, PhD; Kedar Prashant Padhye, MBBS, DNB (Ortho); Narges Rahimee, MD; Anna Ramakrishnan, MS; Saleh Sadeghi, MD; Bernard H. Sagherian, MD, FACS; Jeffrey R. Sawyer, MD; Ran Schwarzkopf, MD, MSc; Webb A. Smith, PhD; Jeyanthi Surendrakumar; Mohamadnaghi Tahmasebi, MD; Kenneth L. Urish, MD, PhD; Jonathan Vigdorchik, MD; William J. Weller, MD; Michael Williams, PT, OCS; Felesfa M. Wodajo, MD; Sandra DeVincent Wolf, PhD; Audrey Zucker-Levin, PhD, PT, MBA.

The planning committee, staff, authors and editors listed below have identified financial relationships or relationships to products or devices they or their spouse/life partner have with commercial interest related to the content of this CME activity:

Judith F. Baumhauer, MD, MPH: is a consultant/advisor for Cartiva

Tyler J. Brolin, MD: is a consultant/advisor for DJO Global.

Emilie Cheung, MD: is a consultant/advisor for Exactech, Inc.

Richard J. Claridge, MD, FRCS: holds a patent/receives royalties with Zimmer Biomet.

Timothy Daniels, MD, FRCSC: is a consultant/advisor for Cartiva.

Mark Glazebrook, MD, PHD, FRCSC: is a consultant/advisor for Cartiva.

Benjamin J. Grear, MD: receives royalties/holds patents with Elsevier.

Adam E. Jakus, PhD: is a shareholder and is employed by Dimensions Inx LLC.

Christopher A. Iobst, MD: is a consultant/advisor for Orthofix Holdings, Inc., NuVasive, Inc., and Smith & Nephew.

William M. Mihalko, MD: participates in a speakers' bureau for Aesculap, Inc. - a B. Braun company and CeramTec GmbH; receives research support from the United States Department of Defense and Stryker; serves as a consultant/advisor for Zimmer Biomet; and receives royalties from Elsevier, Inc.

Patrick C. Toy, MD: has been a consultant/advisor for Zimmer Biomet, Medtronic, and Smith & Nephew. He also receives royalties and/or holds patents with Innomed, Inc.

John C. Weinlein, MD: receives royalties/holds patents with Elsevier, Inc.

UNAPPROVED/OFF-LABEL USE DISCLOSURE

The EOCME requires CME faculty to disclose to the participants:

1. When products or procedures being discussed are off-label, unlabelled, experimental, and/or investigational (not US Food and Drug Administration [FDA] approved); and
2. Any limitations on the information presented, such as data that are preliminary or that represent ongoing research, interim analyses, and/or unsupported opinions. Faculty may discuss information about pharmaceutical agents that is outside of FDA-approved labelling. This information is intended solely for CME and is not intended to promote off-label use of these medications. If you have any questions, contact the medical affairs department of the manufacturer for the most recent prescribing information.

TO ENROLL

To enroll in the *Orthopedic Clinics of North America* Continuing Medical Education program, call customer service at 1-800-654-2452 or sign up online at http://www.theclinics.com/home/cme. The CME program is available to subscribers for an additional annual fee of USD 215.

METHOD OF PARTICIPATION

In order to claim credit, participants must complete the following:

1. Complete enrolment as indicated above.
2. Read the activity.
3. Complete the CME Test and Evaluation. Participants must achieve a score of 70% on the test. All CME Tests and Evaluations must be completed online.

CME INQUIRIES/SPECIAL NEEDS

For all CME inquiries or special needs, please contact elsevierCME@elsevier.com.

EDITORIAL BOARD

CONTRIBUTORS

AUTHORS

YASSER IBRAHIM ALKHALIFE, MBBS, SB
(Orth)
Division of Orthopaedic Surgery, IWK Health
Centre, Halifax, Nova Scotia, Canada

IAN BARRETT, MD
Department of Orthopedic Surgery,
Orthopedic Sports Fellow, Stanford
University, Redwood City, California, USA

JUDITH F. BAUMHAUER, MD, MPH
Professor and Associate Chair of
Orthopaedics, Ortho Department, University
of Rochester School of Medicine and
Dentistry, University of Rochester Medical
Center, Rochester, New York, USA

MICHAEL J. BEEBE, MD
University of Tennessee-Campbell Clinic,
Department of Orthopaedic Surgery and
Biomedical Engineering, Regional One Health,
Memphis, Tennessee, USA

EMILIE CHEUNG, MD
Professor, Department of Orthopedic
Surgery, Stanford University, Redwood City,
California, USA

RICHARD J. CLARIDGE, MD
Assistant Professor, Department of
Orthopaedic Surgery, Mayo Clinic Arizona,
Phoenix, Arizona, USA

TODD K. CONLAN, MD
University of Tennessee-Campbell Clinic,
Department of Orthopaedic Surgery and
Biomedical Engineering, Regional One Health,
Memphis, Tennessee, USA

TIMOTHY DANIELS, MD, FRCSC
Chief, Division of Orthopaedic Surgery, St.
Michaels's Hospital, Professor of Surgery,
University of Toronto, Toronto, Ontario,
Canada

SANDRA DeVINCENT WOLF, PhD
Executive Director, NextManufacturing
Center, Carnegie Mellon University,
Pittsburgh, Pennsylvania, USA

RON EL-HAWARY, MD, MSc, FRCS(C)
Division of Orthopaedic Surgery, IWK Health
Centre, Halifax, Nova Scotia, Canada

AMEER M. ELBULUK, MD
Resident Physician, Hospital for Special
Surgery, New York, New York, USA

REZA A. GHASEMI, MD
Tehran University of Medical Science, Tehran,
Iran

MARK GLAZEBROOK, MD, PhD, FRCSC
Professor of Surgery, Dalhousie University,
Queen Elizabeth II Health Sciences Center,
Halifax Infirmary, Halifax, Nova Scotia, Canada

MATTHEW GOTLIN, MD
Department of Orthopaedic Surgery, Resident
Physician, NYU Langone Orthopedic Hospital,
New York, New York, USA

JAMES G. GURNEY, PhD
Dean, Professor, Division of Epidemiology,
Biostatistics and Environmental Health, School
of Public Health, University of Memphis,
Memphis, Tennessee, USA

CHRISTOPHER A. IOBST, MD
Clinical Associate Professor, Department of
Orthopaedic Surgery, Director, Center for
Limb Lengthening and Reconstruction, The
Ohio State University, College of Medicine,
Nationwide Children's Hospital, Columbus,
Ohio, USA

RICHARD IORIO, MD
Department of Orthopaedic Surgery, Chief,
Adult Reconstruction, Brigham and Women's
Hospital, Boston, Massachusetts, USA

ADAM E. JAKUS, PhD
Chief Technology Officer, Dimension Inx LLC,
Chicago, Illinois, USA

MANESHA LANKACHANDRA, MD
Fellow, Department of Orthopaedics,
MedStar Union Memorial Hospital, Baltimore,
Maryland, USA

MARK LOFTIN, PhD
Associate Dean, School of Applied Sciences,
Professor of Exercise Science, University of
Mississippi, University, Mississippi, USA

WILLIAM M. MIHALKO, MD, PhD
Professor, JR Hyde Chair, Chair, Joint
Graduate Program in Biomedical Engineering,
Director of Adult Reconstructive Fellowship
Program, Department of Orthopedic Surgery
and Biomedical Engineering, Campbell Clinic,
University of Tennessee Health Science
Center, Memphis, Tennessee, USA

PETER N. MITTWEDE, MD, PhD
Resident, Department of Orthopaedic
Surgery, University of Pittsburgh School of
Medicine, Pittsburgh, Pennsylvania, USA

ANAND M. MURTHI, MD
Attending, Department of Orthopaedics,
MedStar Union Memorial Hospital, Baltimore,
Maryland, USA

SNEHA PRABHA NARRA, PhD
Postdoctoral Research Associate,
NextManufacturing Center, College of
Engineering, Carnegie Mellon University,
Pittsburgh, Pennsylvania, USA

DAVID NOVIKOV, BS
Research Assistant, Department of
Orthopaedic Surgery, NYU Langone
Orthopedic Hospital, New York, New York,
USA

KEDAR PRASHANT PADHYE, MBBS, DNB
(Ortho)
Division of Orthopaedic Surgery, IWK Health
Centre, Halifax, Nova Scotia, Canada

NARGES RAHIMEE, MD
Tehran University of Medical Science, Tehran,
Iran

ANNA RAMAKRISHNAN, MS
Clinical Research Assistant, Department of
Orthopedic Surgery, Stanford University,
Redwood City, California, USA

SALEH SADEGHI, MD
Tehran University of Medical Science, Tehran,
Iran

BERNARD H. SAGHERIAN, MD, FACS
Assistant Professor of Clinical Orthopaedic
Surgery, Department of Surgery, Division of
Orthopaedic Surgery, American University of
Beirut Medical Center, Beirut, Lebanon

RAN SCHWARZKOPF, MD, MSc
Department of Orthopaedic Surgery, Associate
Professor, NYU Langone Orthopedic Hospital,
New York, New York, USA

WEBB A. SMITH, PhD
Assistant Professor, Department of Pediatrics,
University of Tennessee Health Science
Center, Memphis, Tennessee, USA

MOHAMADNAGHI TAHMASEBI, MD
Tehran University of Medical Science, Tehran,
Iran

KENNETH L. URISH, MD, PhD
Assistant Professor, Department of
Orthopaedic Surgery, Director, Arthritis
and Arthroplasty Design Group,
Magee-Womens Hospital, Associate
Medical Director, The Bone and Joint Center,
Magee-Womens Hospital, University of
Pittsburgh School of Medicine, Pittsburgh,
Pennsylvania, USA

JONATHAN VIGDORCHIK, MD
Assistant Professor, Department of
Orthopaedic Surgery, NYU Langone
Orthopedic Hospital, New York, New York,
USA

JOHN C. WEINLEIN, MD
University of Tennessee-Campbell Clinic,
Department of Orthopaedic Surgery and
Biomedical Engineering, Regional One Health,
Memphis, Tennessee, USA

WILLIAM J. WELLER, MD
Instructor, Department of Orthopaedic
Surgery and Biomedical Engineering,
University of Tennessee-Campbell Clinic,
Memphis, Tennessee, USA

MICHAEL WILLIAMS, PT, OCS
Director, Department of Physical Therapy,
Campbell Clinic Orthopaedics, Germantown,
Tennessee, USA

FELASFA M. WODAJO, MD
Virginia Cancer Specialists, Fairfax,
Virginia, USA; Associate Professor,
Orthopedic Surgery, VCU School of
Medicine, Richmond, Virginia, USA;
Assistant Professor, Orthopedic Surgery,
Georgetown University Hospital,
Washington, DC, USA

AUDREY ZUCKER-LEVIN, PhD, PT, MBA
GCS Emeritus, Professor, School of Physical
Therapy, College of Medicine, University of
Saskatchewan, Saskatoon, USA

CONTENTS

Knee and Hip Reconstruction
Patrick C. Toy and William M. Mihalko

> Despite the development of newer preventative measures, the rate of infection
> continues to be approximately 1% for patients undergoing total joint arthro-
> plasty (TJA). The extent of the infection can range from a mild superficial infec-
> tion to a more serious periprosthetic joint infection (PJI). PJIs not only play a
> significant role in the clinical well-being of the TJA patient population, but
> also have substantial economic implications on the health care system. Several
> approaches are currently being used to mitigate the risk of PJI after TJA. The
> variety of prophylactic measures to prevent infection after TJA must be thor-
> oughly discussed and evaluated.

> Additive manufacturing (AM) has demonstrated the potential to revolutionize
> manufacturing for various applications across the medical, aerospace, automo-
> bile, and energy sectors. It is a layer-by-layer manufacturing process in which
> the computer-aided design model is sliced into layers and each layer is depos-
> ited successively to realize the final product. This article provides a general
> overview of AM and discusses current state-of-the-art AM methodologies as
> they apply to total joint arthroplasty. Specifically, details on their applications
> and current challenges are summarized to provide orthopedic surgeons with
> a basic understanding of current and potential applications of AM in total joint
> arthroplasty.

> In part 1 of this article, the authors explore nanoscale modifications of the
> surfaces of biomaterials, which offer an exciting potential venue for the pre-
> vention of bacterial adhesion and growth. Despite advances in the design
> and manufacture of implants, infection remains an important and often
> devastating mode of failure. In part 2, additive technologies for tissue engi-
> neering, live cell printing (bioprinting), and tissue fabrication are briefly intro-
> duced. The similarities and differences between bioprinting and non-bio 3D-
> printing approaches and requirements are discussed, along with terminolog-
> ical definitions, current processes, requirements, and biomaterial and cell-
> type selection and sourcing.

Functional limitations persist in obese patients after total knee arthroplasty (TKA). This study assessed the effect of an exercise program (EP) and fitness trackers (FT) in obese patients with TKA. Sixty patients 1 year after orthopedic surgery were recruited and received a 16-week tailored EP; half were randomized to receive an FT. FT had no measurable effect compared with EP alone. EP improved knee range of motion, strength, and quality-of-life scores. This study provides preliminary evidence that a 16-week EP in obese individuals 1 year post TKA is feasible and effective in improving function and quality of life.

Trauma
John C. Weinlein and Michael J. Beebe

This article examines new imaging, diagnostic, and assessment techniques that may affect the care of patients with orthopedic trauma with injury and/or infection. Three-dimensional imaging has assisted in fracture assessment preoperatively, whereas improvement in C-arm technology has allowed real-time evaluation of implant placement and periarticular reduction before leaving the operating room. Advances in imaging techniques have allowed earlier and more accurate diagnosis of nonunion and infection. Innovations in bacteriologic testing have improved the sensitivity and specificity of perioperative and peri-implant infections. It is critical that surgeons remain up to date on the options available for optimal patient care.

Pediatrics
Jeffrey R. Sawyer

Spinal fusion in young children for treatment of early onset scoliosis is not optimal because it limits growth and contributes to long-term lung compromise. Various types of growth-friendly spinal implants and newer technologies have been introduced in the past few years. Similarly, in adolescent idiopathic scoliosis, fusion decreases spinal mobility and may lead to development of adjacent level disc degeneration. A variety of different new technologies have been developed for alternative surgical approaches that halt curve progression while maintaining spinal mobility.

The ability to correct limb deformities is one of the core elements of pediatric orthopedics. The term, orthopedics, is derived from the Greek language and means straightening (*ortho*) children (*paidos*). New advances in the evaluation and management of children with limb alignment or limb length issues are constantly appearing. This review highlights some of the recent technologies that have been developed to improve the care of these children.

Hand and Wrist
Benjamin M. Mauck and James H. Calandruccio

In the field of upper extremity surgery there are myriad new and developing technologies. The purpose of this article is to highlight a few of the most compelling new technologies and review their background, indications for use, and most recently reported outcomes in clinical practice.

Shoulder and Elbow
Tyler J. Brolin

Emerging technologies in shoulder arthroplasty, such as 3-dimensional planning software and real-time intraoperative navigation, are now available for surgeons to perform more accurate placement of the glenoid component without malposition or perforation. Using these tools, the surgeon can visualize the version, inclination, and containment of the implant and determine whether augmented components would be necessary. This review provides an updated investigation of the present literature to elucidate the role of computer navigation in modern shoulder arthroplasty.

Healing rates after rotator cuff repair vary widely. New technologies seek to improve tendon to bone healing with the addition of platelet-rich plasma, stem cells, and biological and synthetic grafts. Platelet-rich plasma and mesenchymal stem cells are used to help create a favorable environment for tendon to bone healing, and grafts and scaffolds provide structural support for repair. The efficacy of platelet-rich plasma and stem cell products seems to be variable, with different products offering different levels of cytokine and growth factors. Scaffold material is also variable with a wide range of synthetic and biological grafts.

Foot and Ankle
Clayton C. Bettin and Benjamin J. Grear

Synthetic cartilage implant surgery is an excellent option for the patient with great toe arthritis and good alignment of the toe who wishes to retain first metatarsophalangeal motion and obtain 90% improved pain relief and function. Patients with osteoporosis, osteopenia, or bone defects from surgery or disease may not maintain the implant position due to poor bone quality, resulting in less than desired outcomes. Despite this being a straightforward surgery, patients need to be aware that the pain relief may not begin until 3+ months after surgery because this procedure does require bone resection and implant placement.

NEW TECHNOLOGIES

SERIES OF RELATED INTEREST

Clinics in Podiatric Medicine and Surgery
Clinics in Sports Medicine
Foot and Ankle Clinics
Hand Clinics
Physical Medicine and Rehabilitation Clinics of North America

PREFACE

New Technologies in Orthopedics

One aspect of orthopedics that makes it such a rewarding and exciting specialty is the continual development of techniques, tools, implants, and other strategies for improving patient outcomes. From Smith-Petersen's glass mold arthroplasty to outpatient joint replacement, additive manufacturing, nanopatterning, and bioprinting—how far total joint arthroplasty (TJA) has come in 100 years! Strategies to prevent periprosthetic infections in TJA are described by Dr Elbuluk and colleagues, who present a variety of prophylactic agents, surgical approaches, and operative techniques developed to mitigate the risk of infection after TJA. Dr Sneha Narra and colleagues provide an excellent overview of additive manufacturing to give us "nontechies" a basic understanding of its applications, and Drs Wodajo and Jakus introduce us to nanoscale modifications of the surfaces of biomaterials that may help prevent bacterial adhesion and growth.

Sometimes, however, new technology doesn't improve the results of old nontechnology. Smith and colleagues studied methods for helping obese patients lose weight and regain motion after total knee arthroplasty (TKA). In their randomized study of the use of exercise and fitness trackers by 60 patients, they found that, while a 4-month exercise program after TKA improved function, the use of a fitness tracker had no measureable effect. Plain old walking worked just as well when it wasn't "tracked."

Dr Conlan and colleagues give us an overview of advances in evaluation and management of trauma patients, including advances in 3D imaging and bacteriologic testing for identifying infecting organisms in perioperative and peri-implant infections, reminding us that it is critical that orthopedic surgeons stay up-to-date on options available.

Two prevalent problems in pediatric patients are spinal and limb deformities, and advances in their management have improved outcomes and quality of life for these patients. As described by Dr Alkhalife and colleagues, alternative surgical approaches, growth-friendly implants, and new technology have lead to techniques that halt scoliosis curve progression while maintaining spinal mobility. Dr Iobst reviews the recent technologies designed to improve the care of children with limb alignment or limb length issues.

Dr Weller gives an overview of the myriad of new and developing technologies for upper extremity surgery, including new implants for thumb carpometacarpal arthroplasty and nerve allografts and conduits for digital nerve repairs. The review by Dr Barrett and colleagues provides an updated investigation of the present literature to further define the role of computer navigation in modern shoulder arthroplasty, while Drs Murthi and Lankachandra describe the use of technologies such as platelet-rich plasma and mesenchymal stem cells to improve tendon-to-bone healing in rotator cuff repair.

Several reconstructive procedures in foot and ankle surgery require structural grafts to fill defects, restore height, and maintain correction until fusion occurs. Newer options include synthetic cartilage implants, as described by Dr Baumhauer and colleagues, and tantalum metal implants, as described by Drs Sagherian and Claridge. Bone marrow edema syndrome is a rare and self-limited syndrome with an unknown cause. Dr Ghasemi and colleagues introduce us to this entity and review its diagnosis using MRI and ultrasound and its treatment with physical modalities, pharmaceuticals, and surgery.

We hope you will be as intrigued as we are with all the new technology described in this issue.

Frederick M. Azar, MD
Campbell Clinic
University of Tennessee–Campbell Clinic
Department of Orthopaedic Surgery
1211 Union Avenue, Suite 510
Memphis, TN 38104, USA

E-mail address:
fazar@campbellclinic.com

https://doi.org/10.1016/j.ocl.2018.09.001
0030-5898/19/© 2018 Published by Elsevier Inc.

Knee and Hip Reconstruction

Control Strategies for Infection Prevention in Total Joint Arthroplasty

Ameer M. Elbuluk, MD[a],*, David Novikov, BS[b],
Matthew Gotlin, MD[b], Ran Schwarzkopf, MD, MSc[b],
Richard Iorio, MD[c], Jonathan Vigdorchik, MD[b]

KEYWORDS
• Total joint arthroplasty • Infection • Hip • Knee • Outcomes

KEY POINTS
• Periprosthetic joint infection remains one of the most common and costly complications after total joint arthroplasty (TJA).   • Infection control is an important consideration in all surgical procedures, but especially in TJA, which incorporates foreign implants and can result in costly revisions.   • This article highlights the importance of preoperative, intraoperative, and postoperative infection control measures and helps to serve as a framework to weigh the pros and cons of interventions at each stage of surgical management.

INTRODUCTION

Infection remains one of the most frequent and expensive complications after total joint arthroplasty (TJA).[1] It is currently the leading cause of revision total knee arthroplasty (TKA) and the third most common cause of revision total hip arthroplasty (THA) in the United States.[2,3] Despite the development of several preventative measures, the rate of infection continues to affect approximately 1% of patients undergoing TKA and THA.[4] Infections can range from a minor superficial infection to a more serious periprosthetic joint infection (PJI).

In addition to the significant clinical impact that PJIs have on the TJA patient population, there are also major economic implications for the health care system. Infection results in increased length of stay (LOS), increased readmission rates, and increased need for medical interventions.[5,6] TKA and THA frequency is projected to increase by 673% and 174%, respectively, by 2030. Therefore, limiting complications such as PJI will be paramount to maintaining the viability of these procedures.[7]

Currently, many different strategies are used to mitigate the risk of PJI after TJA and newer approaches are constantly in development. Accordingly, the variety of prophylactic agents and/or protocols created to prevent infection after TJA must be thoroughly evaluated. For the purpose of discussion, these agents and/or protocols can be divided into preoperative, intraoperative, and postoperative measures. This review thoroughly examines the opportunities for infection prevention during each of these transitions of care.

Disclosure Statement: None.
[a] Hospital for Special Surgery, 535 East 70th Street, New York, NY 10021, USA; [b] Department of Orthopaedic Surgery, NYU Langone Orthopedic Hospital, 301 East 17th Street, New York, NY 10003, USA; [c] Department of Orthopaedic Surgery, Adult Reconstruction, Brigham and Women's Hospital, 60 Fenwood Road, Boston, MA 02115, USA
* Corresponding author.
E-mail address: elbulukam@hss.edu

PREOPERATIVE

Methicillin-Resistant *Staphylococcus aureus* and *Staphyloccocus* Screening and Decolonization

Staphylococcus aureus is the organism found to have the highest association with surgical site infection (SSI) after TJA. It has been reported to colonize the nasal area in approximately 33% of the population.[8–10] As such, many studies have examined the impact of minimizing the colonization and population density of both methicillin-sensitive *S aureus* and methicillin-resistant *S aureus* (MRSA) in patients undergoing TJA.

A systematic review by Chen and colleagues[11] examined 19 studies that evaluated the effectiveness of various *S aureus* decolonization protocols in their ability to reduce SSI in patients undergoing TJA. Each study substantiated the evidence that *S aureus* screening and decolonization (with the use of mupirocin alone or in combination of other agents) was an effective means of reducing SSI.[11] Furthermore, these models also showed that implementing an *S aureus* decolonization protocol was an economically preferred strategy compared with a nontreatment group. For example, Courville and colleagues[12] demonstrated a savings of $330 per quality-adjusted life year in THA and $438 saved per quality-adjusted life year for TKA when all patients were decolonized compared with a nontreatment group.

As intranasal screening and treatment have become more widespread, however, the benefits of these screening programs must be carefully weighed against the economic and clinical implications of implementing a routine screening and decolonization program. In a retrospective evaluation, Torres and colleagues[13] compared the universal administration of povidone-iodine nasal swabs to MRSA screening and subsequent treatment in 1853 TJA patients to determine their impact on the incidence of SSI at 90 days. The investigators found that patients who did not undergo MRSA screening and received a povidone-iodine swab and chlorhexidine bath for 5 days leading up to surgery had similar rates of infection (0.8%) as patients who were screened and treated for MRSA with a 5-day course of mupirocin and chlorhexidine bath prior to surgery (0.8%). This povidone-iodine protocol also allowed for an average cost savings of $93.35 per patient ($P<.01$).[13] Thus, although screening and decolonization protocols have a certain level of clinical and economic benefit, the universal povidone-iodine protocol may provide equal infection control and be more cost effective.

Chlorhexidine Skin Preparation

Preoperative whole-body bathing, showering, or skin cleansing with chlorhexidine gluconate (CHG), a topical antiseptic, has been shown to reduce native skin flora and in effect limit the risk of SSIs and health care–associated infections postoperatively.[14,15] Moreover, CHG is an affordable option believed to have minimal side effects. Although rare cases of anaphylaxis have been reported, side effects are typically limited to localized skin reactions.[16] Studies have documented significantly decreased SSI risk when TJA patients are compliant with the CHG protocol.[17,18] In a prospective consecutive series, Johnson and colleagues[18] found that patients who used CHG wipes 1 day prior to THA and on the morning of their operation had a lower incidence of SSI (0%) than patients who did not comply (1.6% infection rate) with this protocol (patients with partial compliance were excluded). Similar results were reported in a prospective, randomized controlled trial by Kapadia and colleagues.[17] The investigators found a lower rate of PJI at 1-year follow-up in a cohort of TJA patients who used a CHG cloth the night before and day of surgery compared with to a cohort of patients who bathed with soap and water prior to[19] surgery (0.4% vs 2.9%; $P<.05$).[17] Another study by Kapadia and colleagues[20] examined 2458 patients undergoing THA and evaluated whether preadmission cutaneous CHG preparations compared with a standard in-hospital perioperative preparation (0.7% iodine povacrylex and 74% isopropyl alcohol) reduced SSI. Overall, they found that the use of a preoperative CHG cloth skin preparation was associated with a reduced relative risk (RR) of SSI after THA compared with patients undergoing in-hospital perioperative skin preparation only (3/557, or 0.5%, compared with 32/1901, or 1.7%; $P = .04$).[20]

When comparing to skin cleansing with CHG soap and baths, recent reports show that CHG infused clothes are more effective because they have higher antiseptic cutaneous concentrations. Edmiston and colleagues[19] found that a 2% CHG cloth had a 12.7-times to 27.4-times higher mean skin CHG concentration than a shower with 4% CHG soap at all cutaneous sites ($P<.001$). The cost-effectiveness of using CHG cloth preparations as an infection prevention tool has also been evaluated. In an epidemiologic study by Kapadia and colleagues,[21] a cost-benefit analysis of the addition of a preoperative CHG cloth preparation per 1000 patients undergoing TKA at their institution revealed an annual net savings of $2.1 million.

The effectiveness of CHG in reducing SSI has been challenged, however, by Chlebicki and colleagues.[22] In a meta-analysis of 16 clinical trials comparing a total of 17,932 patients, the investigators demonstrated no significant reduction in the overall incidence of SSI when CHG was compared with soap, placebo, or no shower/bathing (RR 0.9; CI, 0.77–1.05; P = .19). Although the investigators concede that many of the included studies had suboptimal designs, this study sheds light on the need for higher-quality randomized clinical trials to fully elucidate the potential benefit of CHG.[22] Nonetheless, as a relatively affordable and low-risk treatment, even a marginal clinical benefit may justify its use.

Antibiotic Stewardship and Dual Antibiotics

Several clinical studies have shown the added benefit of parenteral prophylactic antibiotics in decreasing the likelihood of SSIs.[23,24] The preferred routine antibiotic agent for TJA recipients has generally been cefazolin, a first-generation cephalosporin that helps suppress staphylococcal dermal and incisional infections. Its recommended dose is 1.0 g for patients who weigh less than 80 kg and 2.0 g for those who weigh greater than 80 kg.[25] Additionally, it should be completely infused within 1 hour prior to skin incision to reach optimal tissue concentration.[25] It is effective against gram-positive organisms as well as a majority of clinically relevant aerobic gram-negative bacilli (GNB) and has been found to distribute well in bone, muscle, and synovium.[26] Since its adoption as the prophylactic agent of choice in the 1960s, however, there has been little to no change to preoperative prophylactic regimens. Furthermore, cefazolin may be inadequate at some institutions because of high rates of MRSA and GNB. For instance, a study by Norton and colleagues[27] demonstrated that 30% of SSIs after THA were actually caused by GNB.

Due to increasing antibiotic resistance and presence of GNB, Bosco and colleagues[28] studied the effect of Expanded Gram-Negative Antimicrobial Prophylaxis (EGNAP) on SSI rates after primary TJA. To expand gram-negative antimicrobial prophylaxis, their institution added weight-based high-dose gentamicin (or aztreonam if gentamicin was contraindicated) to their prophylactic antibiotic protocol for TJA patients. In this study, there were 10,084 cases; THA and TKA accounted for 5389 and 4695 cases, respectively. Before the introduction of EGNAP, SSI rates in THA patients were 1.19% (49/4122). After July 2012, when EGNAP was added, the overall SSI rates in THA patients decreased to 0.55% (7/1267; P = .05). During the study period, however, there was no significant difference in SSI rates among TKA patients: 1.08% versus 1.02% (P = .999). In addition to decreasing GNB SSIs with gentamicin or aztreonam, there was also a significant decrease in gram-positive bacteria SSIs from 1.01% (41/4122) to 0.47% (6/1267) (P = .05). Their study demonstrated that the addition of high-dose weight-based gentamicin or aztreonam prophylaxis for hip arthroplasty is a safe and effective method to decrease SSIs.

Another study by Sewick and colleagues,[29] however, examined whether dual antibiotic prophylaxis (1) reduced the rate of SSI compared with single antibiotic prophylaxis and (2) altered the microbiology of SSI in patients undergoing TJA. They retrospectively reviewed 1828 primary THAs and TKAs and divided patients into 2 groups: (1) those who received a dual prophylactic antibiotic regimen of cefazolin and vancomycin (unless allergic) and (2) those who received cefazolin (unless allergic) as the sole prophylactic antibiotic. The infection rates for dual antibiotic prophylaxis compared with a single antibiotic regimen were 1.1% and 1.4%, respectively. Their study concluded that the addition of vancomycin as a prophylactic antibiotic agent did not significantly reduce the rate of SSI compared with cefazolin alone (P = .636) but could reduce the incidence of MRSA infections (0.08% vs 0.8%; P = .022).[29] These results support recommendations to limit the use of vancomycin prophylaxis to only known MRSA-positive cases in an effort to minimize the development of vancomycin-resistant enterococci and MRSA.[30]

Bacterial resistance patterns continue to evolve and influence antibiotic prescription practices. As a result, antibiotic stewardship programs (ASPs) that consist of a multidisciplinary team of surgeons, clinical pharmacists, infectious disease specialists, and infection control practitioners were created. These teams monitor antimicrobial use and make recommendations based on the prevalence of infecting organisms in an effort to use the best empiric therapy.[31] The utility of ASPs has been supported, with some studies showing a 36% increase in the infection cure rate and a 26% decrease in the failure rate at a single institution after it instituted an ASP.[32] ASPs take into account information, such as the microbial landscape, at any given institution when making antibiotic regimen recommendations. Furthermore, ASPs use the use of molecular assays to create antibiograms, or databases of local bacterial organisms and their antimicrobial susceptibilities, that can help providers tailor and individualize empiric therapy through the monitoring of antimicrobial resistance.[31,33]

The American Academy of Orthopaedic Surgeons (AAOS) has recommended the use of vancomycin as a prophylactic agent for TJA recipients at institutions with a high prevalence (ie, >10%–20%) of MRSA.[34,35] A study by Smith and colleagues[36] demonstrated the successful transition from cefazolin to vancomycin as a prophylactic antibiotic to combat their increasing MRSA burden. The investigators were able to significantly reduce their total PJI rate from 1% to 0.5% (P = .03) and their MRSA PJI rate from 0.23% to 0.07% (P = .14) over a 4-year period.

These studies highlight the importance of establishing a robust institutional SSI surveillance and ASP. In hospitals with organisms that are resistant to standard cephalosporin-based prophylactic regimens, such as MRSA or GNB, these programs can help elucidate the evolving patterns and virulence of these resistant pathogens as well as tailor more effective surgical prophylaxis.

Patient Risk Factor Modification/ Optimization

The AAOS has identified several modifiable risk factors (MRFs) for the development of SSI in TJA patients.[30] MRFs are defined as risk factors that potentially could be corrected, optimized, or treated.[37] Previously reported MRFs that increase the risk for PJI after TJA include obesity,[38] malnutrition,[39] diabetes,[38] preoperative anemia,[40] HIV,[39] S aureus colonization,[38] depression,[41] and tobacco use.[42] Moucha and colleagues[42] found that among TJA candidates at their institution, 80% were patients with MRFs. Considering TJA is an elective procedure, preoperative patient optimization and delay of surgery in appropriate patients can help decrease infection and improve outcomes. Numerous studies have demonstrated that obesity is associated with an increased risk for SSI after TJA.[25,43–45] Although there is no clear body mass index (BMI) cutoff, reports suggest that BMIs greater than 40 kg/m^2 are significantly associated with SSI (P<.007).[37,43] A study by Namba and colleagues[46] showed that the risk for infection is 6.7-times and 4.2-times higher in obese patients undergoing TKA and THA, respectively. Obese patients were more likely to have longer surgical times (odds ratio [OR] 1.211; 95% CI, 1.169–1.255),[45] experience prolonged postoperative wound drainage

(TKA: P = .584; THA: P = .054),[47] increased blood loss (30%–67% increase in transfusions), diets lacking in essential vitamins and minerals,[39] and comorbid conditions such as diabetes.[39] Counseling patients on various weight loss strategies, including bariatric surgery, is encouraged. Rapid weight loss prior to surgery, however, places patients at risk of a catabolic state and malnutrition, ultimately predisposing them to complications.[46,48] If a patient chooses to undergo bariatric surgery, adequate time for weight loss and medical comorbidity optimization theoretically is needed. Schwarzkopf and colleagues[49] were among the first to retrospectively analyze the correlation between time from bariatric surgery and outcomes after TJA. They demonstrated that THA recipients were more less likely to be readmitted if their arthroplasty surgery was done greater than 6 months after bariatric surgery. They failed to find any association, however, between time from bariatric surgery to TJA and respective complication rates. Although the data showed that it may be beneficial to wait 6 months after bariatric surgery to undergo THA, the investigators were unable to make any definitive recommendations.

Nutritional optimization enhances patients' ability to suppress the growth of foreign pathogens and minimizes their risk for PJI. Patients who are at risk for malnutrition, including the elderly and patients with gastrointestinal disease, renal disease, alcoholism, and cancer, should undergo a nutritional evaluation prior to TJA.[39] Studies have shown that lymphocyte counts greater than 1500 cells/μL, albumin levels greater than 3.5 g/dL, zinc levels greater than 5 μg/dL, and transferrin levels greater than 200 mg/dL can decrease the risk of superficial infection, delayed wound healing, and PJI.[30] Therefore, nutritional supplementation based on a patients' individualized assessment can help optimize their nutritional status and minimize their risk for infection.

Diabetes, defined as a chronic disease diagnosed by fasting blood sugar levels greater than 126 mg/dL and/or hemoglobin A$_{1c}$ greater than 6.5% on 2 separate occasions, has been identified as an independent MRF for PJI in TJA patients.[50,51] With an estimated 8% of TJA patients identified as diabetic[52] and an approximate 4-fold greater risk for infection (3.4% vs 0.86%; P<.001), optimization of this MRF is imperative.[53,54] Although the American Diabetes Association recommends keeping hemoglobin A$_{1c}$ levels less than 7% prior to surgery, studies have failed to validate this cutoff and its predictive ability for infection in TJA patients.[54] Alternatively, hyperglycemia, as measured by perioperative serum glucose levels, has been reported to be a more reliable predictor of infection in TJA patients (hazard ratio 1.44; $P<.008$), making it a potential target for optimization.[55] Jamsen and colleagues[53] reported that glucose levels less than 100 mg/dL correlated with a 1-year infection rate of 0.44%, whereas glucose levels greater than 125 mg/dL correlated with an infection of 2.42%. It has been postulated that hyperglycemia impairs various immune system functions that defend against bacteria, thus predisposing the patient to infection.[56] Hyperglycemia can result from surgical stress or from underlying uncontrolled diabetes.[55] Therefore, through coordination with primary care providers, preoperative glycemic testing and tight glycemic control are essential to improving outcomes. Goals of fasting glucose less than 180 mg/dL, nonfasting glucose less than 200 mg/dL, and hemoglobin A_{1c} less than 8% have been reported in the literature.[57]

With improvements in the management of patients with HIV, an increasing number of HIV-positive patients are living long enough to develop degenerative arthritis requiring TJA.[58,59] Furthermore, HIV-positive patients are 100-times more likely to develop osteonecrosis, a direct result of the infection and from various treatment modalities, including corticosteroids and protease inhibitors.[58,60] Considering CD4 counts less than 200 cells/mm^3 or viral loads greater than 10,000 copies/mL are associated with an increased incidence of complications, preoperative coordination with infectious disease specialists in an effort to strengthen a patient's immune system is vital to reduce risk of infection.[39]

Lastly, it has long been established that tobacco use and smoking adversely affect postoperative outcomes and are substantial risk factors for poor wound healing (OR 3.2; $P = .001$)[61] and infection (OR 1.47; $P<.05$).[62] Nicotine causes microvascular vasoconstriction whereas carbon monoxide binds to hemoglobin, forming carboxyhemoglobin, subsequently leading to tissue hypoxia.[63,64] Considering approximately 7% of TJA patients are current tobacco users,[65] tobacco cessation protocols have been widely adopted.[66,67] Current recommendations advocate for smoking cessation 4 weeks to 8 weeks prior to elective TJA, because studies have shown a 65% reduction in postoperative complications.[67] Preoperative screening for smoking can include a patient-reported self-assessment and/or a biochemical analysis of cotinine (nicotine metabolite) or exhaled carbon monoxide.[68]

INTRAOPERATIVE
Irrigation Techniques
Intraoperative wound irrigation is common practice despite a lack of standardization among orthopedic surgeons.[69] Irrigation with 0.9% saline, antibiotic solutions, and povidone-iodine lavages has been reported. In a retrospective study by Brown and colleagues,[70] the investigators evaluated the effectiveness of an infection prevention protocol consisting of dilute Betadine lavage prior to wound closure in TJA. Betadine, a combination of povidone and iodine, is a chemical solution that releases free iodine and is toxic to microorganisms. The Betadine solution they used consisted of povidone-iodine mixed with 500 mL of sterile isotonic sodium chloride, resulting in a 0.35% povidone-iodine solution.[70] The surgeon would soak the wound with 500 mL of dilute Betadine for 3 minutes after implantation of the prosthetic components. This was followed by pulsatile lavage with 1 L of isotonic sodium chloride and application of 10% Betadine to the skin surrounding the incision just prior to closure. The investigators compared this modified protocol to a previous one, which consisted of lavage with 1 L of isotonic sodium chloride only. This modified protocol resulted in a significantly lower rate of infection after TJA (0.97% vs 0.15%; $P = .04$).[70] Given the low cost ($1.11 per Betadine packet) and minimal side-effect profile, the investigators concluded that the use of this irrigation protocol was safe and inexpensive. Conversely, others have found that the use of Betadine is associated with chondrocyte toxicity. von Keudell and colleagues[71] analyzed the effect of povidone-iodine solutions on bovine cartilage and found increasing rates of cell death within the superficial cartilage layer when it was exposed to this solution. Although not applicable to TJA, this chondrotoxicity can adversely affect partial arthroplasty or TKA without resurfacing.[71]

More recently, Frisch and colleagues[72] reported on the addition of 0.05% CHG solution to intraoperative saline irrigation in TJA. The investigators found no difference in SSI when they compared the use of a newer protocol, consisting of intraoperative irrigation with 0.9% saline and recurrent 0.05% CHG lavage, with an older protocol consisting of 0.9% saline followed by dilute povidone-iodine washout in THA, and 0.9% saline as a sole agent in TKA. They attributed the lack of significance to the underpowered nature and low sample size of the study.[72] Future studies are needed to evaluate the effectiveness and safety of povidone-iodone and

CHG irrigation as a combined infection prevention method tool.

Wound Closure

Given the emphasis on rapid rehabilitation and shorter LOS, the optimal method of wound closure should maximize skin healing, minimize dehiscence, and decrease infection.[73] The most common methods of skin closure are metal staples, sutures, and less frequently adhesives.[74] A wide variety of suture materials are used, such as barbed, braided, monofilament, absorbable, nonabsorbable, and synthetic sutures. Adhesives include materials, such as 2-octylcyanoacrylate (OCA), or super glue.[75,76] A recent meta-analysis by Kim and colleagues[77] evaluated differences in complications, including deep and superficial infections, between skin closure with sutures or staples in TKA procedures. Results demonstrated a higher risk for superficial infection (RR 1.78; $P = .22$), deep infection (RR 3.78; $P = .91$), and wound dehiscence (RR 1.63; $P = .22$) with sutures compared with staples, although the results failed to reach significance. Conversely, the investigators found that skin closure with sutures resulted in a lower risk for prolonged wound drainage (RR 0.48; $P = .76$); however, the results were also not statistically significant. The investigators concluded that staple closure carries a few subtle advantages over suture closure in TKA, albeit the investigators mentioned that more studies are required to definitively establish superiority.[77]

In another randomized controlled trial by Khan and colleagues,[75] the investigators demonstrated no significant difference between the use of subcuticular suture (Monocryl), OCA, and staples in regard to infection after TJA. The investigators concluded that skin closure with staples was significantly faster ($P<.0001$) and thus superior to the other 2 techniques. Conversely, a meta-analysis by Smith and colleagues[73] found that the risk of developing a superficial wound infection was 3-times greater when wounds were closed with metal staples compared with sutures in TJA patients (RR 3.83; $P = .01$). A follow-up study to this meta-analysis by Krishnan and colleagues[78] found conflicting results as they demonstrated no difference in infection rates between skin closures with sutures compared with staples (RR 1.06; $P>.05$).

Livesey and colleagues[74] conducted a randomized controlled trial comparing skin closure with the use of a LiquiBand surgical skin adhesive with surgical staples in THA procedures and demonstrated no difference in complication rates ($P = .3$). Additionally, they found that mean time for closure with staples was faster (70.5 seconds vs 181.6 seconds; $P = .002$) and that staples were more cost-effective to use than the skin adhesive (7.63USD vs 25.83USD).

A more recent addition to the myriad closure methods is barbed suture. This suture does not require knots and has been demonstrated to approximate edges of tissue quicker than traditional suturing and with the use of less material.[76] A retrospective study evaluating clinical outcomes with the use of barbed suture compared with metallic staples for superficial wound closure in TKA patients found that barbed suture had a higher incidence of superficial infection (11.8% vs 3.2%; $P = .002$) and deep infection (4.7% vs 0.8%; $P = .0128$).[76] In both groups, the arthrotomy was closed with polyglyconate suture. The results of the study prompted the investigators to discontinue the use of barbed suture for closure in TKA.[76]

As evidenced by the aforementioned conflicting results, the best method for closure is still under debate and should be further explored through adequately powered clinical trials in the future. Additionally, many surgeons use a combined approach to wound closure (eg, Monocryl plus adhesives); therefore, future studies evaluating the efficacy and cost-effectiveness of this strategy are warranted.

Vancomycin Powder

The use of vancomycin powder has yet to be validated in TJA. Several studies, however, have shown a decreased incidence of deep wound infections with the local use of vancomycin during spine and trauma procedures.[79–82] Schroeder and colleagues[83] examined the use of vancomycin powder into surgical wounds prior to closing of the fascia as a method to reduce deep infection rates in 1224 patients undergoing spine procedures. Their study found 30 cases of deep infections needing a surgical irrigation and débridement without vancomycin versus 5 when vancomycin was used ($P = .04$). Infections in patients treated with vancomycin did not involve vancomycin-resistant bacteria. The number needed to treat to reduce 1 case of deep infection in this study was approximately 200. Despite this large number, treatment with local vancomycin has been shown to be a cost-effective measure compared with the high costs associated with care of deep infections.

Wukich and colleagues[84] also examined the efficacy of local vancomycin powder to reduce SSI in patients with diabetes mellitus (DM) undergoing foot and ankle surgery. Eighty-one patients with DM who underwent reconstructive surgery due to a foot and/or ankle deformity and/or trauma received topically applied vancomycin. These patients were matched to 81 with DM who did not receive topically applied vancomycin. The 2 groups were similar with regard to gender, BMI, duration of DM, short-term and longer-term glycemic control, and length of surgery. The overall likelihood of SSI was decreased by 73% in patients who received topically applied vancomycin (OR 0.27; P = .019). Although the rate of superficial infection was not significantly different between the 2 groups (OR 0.400; P = .27), deep infections were 80% less likely in patients who received vancomycin powder (OR 0.200; P = .04). They found that high-risk diabetic patients undergoing foot and ankle surgery were notably less likely to develop an SSI with the use of topically applied vancomycin powder in the surgical wound, in particular deep infections. Concerning costs, topically applied vancomycin powder was inexpensive ($5 per 1000 mg) and associated with a very low rate of complications, thus reducing potential downstream costs. Based on this study, they conclude that foot and ankle surgeons may consider applying 500 mg to 1000 mg of vancomycin powder prior to skin closure in diabetic patients who are not allergic to vancomycin.

The efficacy of vancomycin powder in reducing SSI in other areas of orthopedics is promising; however, its use in TJA as a tool to decrease SSI still needs to be validated.

POSTOPERATIVE
Wound Dressings

Wound dressings provide a protective barrier that is critical for minimizing contamination and promoting healing after surgery. When managing a wound, a moist occlusive wound environment has been found to be favorable to a dry wound environment by limiting desiccation and cellular death.[85–88] Such an environment, however, can also increase the risk of microbial colonization if not properly managed. Therefore, the most effective wound dressings must maintain a moist environment while protecting the incision area from contamination and further damage.

Multiple dressing types have been developed toward achieving this goal. Currently, literature discussing wound dressing use after TJA relates mainly to the use of hydrofiber dressings, such as Aquacel and Aquacel Ag (ConvaTec, Bridgewater, New Jersey).[44,89–93] Hydrofiber wound dressings are composed of sodium carboxymethyl cellulose and help maintain a moist

environment, allowing for fewer dressing changes with improved wound healing.[94–96] Silver impregnated Aquacel (Aquacel Ag) is similar to the generic Aquacel dressings, except that it also contains ionic silver that acts as a bacteriostatic agent.[89,90,94] Studies by Cai and colleagues[90] and Grosso and colleagues[89] have demonstrated strong evidence supporting the use of hydrofiber dressing, such as Aquacel Ag, compared with other dressings. Grosso and colleagues[89] reviewed 1173 consecutive charts of patients undergoing TJA and found that the Aquacel Ag group had a significantly decreased rate of PJI (0.33%) compared with the standard sterile xeroform dressings (1.58%). According to a retrospective review by Cai and colleagues[90] of 903 consecutive subjects who received Aquacel dressings and 875 cases who received standard dressings, the prevalence of acute PJI was significantly lower in the Aqaucel group (0.44% vs 1.71%). Together these studies highlight the potential for infection reduction through the use of Aquacel dressings. From the Cai and colleagues[90] study, if Aquacel dressings were to be used routinely after TJA in the United States, this would add approximately $27 million in cost. If these figures are correct, however, then the additional cost may be balanced with the savings from reduced readmissions, LOS, and other factors related to management of infection after TJA.

This premise has been challenged by at least 1 study, by Ubbink and colleagues,[97] that compared occlusive, moist-environment dressings to standard gauze-based dressings and found no significant difference in time to complete wound healing. Although this study did not look at hydrofiber dressings alone in the occlusive group, it highlights an important consideration in infection prevention. These studies demonstrate the need for more robust literature to evaluate the effectiveness of hydrofiber dressings before they can be widely used for all TJA patients.

SUMMARY

Infection control is an important consideration in all surgical procedures, but especially in TJA, which incorporates foreign implants and can result in costly revisions. Multiple opportunities exist to improve intraoperative, perioperative, and postoperative infection control (Table 1). Accordingly, each discussed intervention must be carefully evaluated to determine its value in preventing this significant complication. Ultimately, this review highlights the importance of infection prevention and can serve as a

Table 1
Summary of recommendations for infection prevention in total joint arthroplasty

Perioperative Stage	Factor	Recommendation
Preoperative	MRSA and *Staphylococcus* screening and decolonization	Consider universal use of povidone-iodine nasal swab prior to surgery regardless of MRSA status
	Chlorhexidine skin preparation	CHG wipe use 1 day prior and on the morning of surgery
	Antibiotic stewardship and dual antibiotics	• Prophylactic use of first-generation cephalosporin and weight-based gentamicin or aztreonam 1 hour prior to skin incision • At institutions with a high prevalence of MRSA (>10%–20%), vancomycin as a prophylactic agent is recommended • Antibiotic stewardship and surveillance programs can help tailor more effective surgical prophylaxis
	Patient risk factor modification/optimization	Optimize MRFs (obesity, diabetes, HIV, and tobacco use) using a multidisciplinary approach prior to TJA
Intraoperative	Irrigation techniques	Consider using a dilute Betadine lavage prior to wound closure
	Wound closure	Evidence is inconclusive
	Vancomycin powder	Currently not validated for use in TJA; however, results are promising in spine and trauma surgeries
Postoperative	Wound dressings	Promising results have been demonstrated with use of Aquacel dressings despite their cost

framework to help weigh the pros and cons of each stage of surgical management.

REFERENCES

1. Lindeque B, Hartman Z, Noshchenko A, et al. Infection after primary total hip arthroplasty. Orthopedics 2014;37:257–65.
2. Bozic KJ, Kurtz SM, Lau E, et al. The epidemiology of revision total knee arthroplasty in the United States. Clin Orthop Relat Res 2010;468:45–51.
3. Bozic KJ, Kurtz SM, Lau E, et al. The epidemiology of revision total hip arthroplasty in the United States. J Bone Joint Surg Am 2009;91:128–33.
4. Kurtz SM, Lau E, Schmier J, et al. Infection burden for hip and knee arthroplasty in the United States. J Arthroplasty 2008;23:984–91.
5. Bozic KJ, Ries MD. The impact of infection after total hip arthroplasty on hospital and surgeon resource utilization. J Bone Joint Surg Am 2005; 87:1746–51.
6. Sculco TP. The economic impact of infected joint arthroplasty. Orthopedics 1995;18:871–3.
7. Kurtz S, Ong K, Lau E, et al. Projections of primary and revision hip and knee arthroplasty in the United States from 2005 to 2030. J Bone Joint Surg Am 2007;89:780–5.
8. Ramos N, Stachel A, Phillips M, et al. Prior Staphylococcus aureus nasal colonization: a risk factor for surgical site infections following decolonization. J Am Acad Orthop Surg 2016;24:880–5.
9. Mainous AG 3rd, Hueston WJ, Everett CJ, et al. Nasal carriage of Staphylococcus aureus and methicillin-resistant S aureus in the United States, 2001-2002. Ann Fam Med 2006;4:132–7.
10. Wertheim HF, Melles DC, Vos MC, et al. The role of nasal carriage in Staphylococcus aureus infections. Lancet Infect Dis 2005;5:751–62.
11. Chen AF, Wessel CB, Rao N. Staphylococcus aureus screening and decolonization in orthopaedic surgery and reduction of surgical site infections. Clin Orthop Relat Res 2013;471:2383–99.
12. Courville XF, Tomek IM, Kirkland KB, et al. Cost-effectiveness of preoperative nasal mupirocin treatment in preventing surgical site infection in patients undergoing total hip and knee arthroplasty:

a cost-effectiveness analysis. Infect Control Hosp Epidemiol 2012;33:152–9.

13. Torres EG, Lindmair-Snell JM, Langan JW, et al. Is preoperative nasal povidone-iodine as efficient and cost-effective as standard methicillin-resistant Staphylococcus aureus screening protocol in total joint arthroplasty? J Arthroplasty 2016;31:215–8.

14. Schweizer ML, Chiang HY, Septimus E, et al. Association of a bundled intervention with surgical site infections among patients undergoing cardiac, hip, or knee surgery. JAMA 2015;313:2162–71.

15. Edmiston CE, Krepel CJ, Spencer MP, et al. Preadmission application of 2% chlorhexidine gluconate (CHG): enhancing patient compliance while maximizing skin surface concentrations. Infect Control Hosp Epidemiol 2016;37:254–9.

16. Abbas S, Sastry S. Chlorhexidine: patient bathing and infection prevention. Curr Infect Dis Rep 2016;18:25.

17. Kapadia BH, Elmallah RK, Mont MA. A randomized, clinical trial of preadmission chlorhexidine skin preparation for lower extremity total joint arthroplasty. J Arthroplasty 2016;31:2856–61.

18. Johnson AJ, Daley JA, Zywiel MG, et al. Preoperative chlorhexidine preparation and the incidence of surgical site infections after hip arthroplasty. J Arthroplasty 2010;25:98–102.

19. Edmiston CE Jr, Krepel CJ, Seabrook GR, et al. Preoperative shower revisited: can high topical antiseptic levels be achieved on the skin surface before surgical admission? J Am Coll Surg 2008; 207:233–9.

20. Kapadia BH, Johnson AJ, Daley JA, et al. Preadmission cutaneous chlorhexidine preparation reduces surgical site infections in total hip arthroplasty. J Arthroplasty 2013;28:490–3.

21. Kapadia BH, Johnson AJ, Issa K, et al. Economic evaluation of chlorhexidine cloths on healthcare costs due to surgical site infections following total knee arthroplasty. J Arthroplasty 2013;28:1061–5.

22. Chlebicki MP, Safdar N, O'Horo JC, et al. Preoperative chlorhexidine shower or bath for prevention of surgical site infection: a meta-analysis. Am J Infect Control 2013;41:167–73.

23. Burke JF. The effective period of preventive antibiotic action in experimental incisions and dermal lesions. Surgery 1961;50:161–8.

24. Oishi CS, Carrion WV, Hoaglund FT. Use of parenteral prophylactic antibiotics in clean orthopaedic surgery. A review of the literature. Clin Orthop Relat Res 1993;(296):249–55.

25. Pulido L, Ghanem E, Joshi A, et al. Periprosthetic joint infection: the incidence, timing, and predisposing factors. Clin Orthop Relat Res 2008;466:1710–5.

26. Neu HC. Cephalosporin antibiotics as applied in surgery of bones and joints. Clin Orthop Relat Res 1984;(190):50–64.

27. Norton TD, Skeete F, Dubrovskaya Y, et al. Orthopedic surgical site infections: analysis of causative bacteria and implications for antibiotic stewardship. Am J Orthop (Belle Mead NJ) 2014;43:E89–92.

28. Bosco JA, Prince Rainier RT, Catanzano AJ, et al. Expanded gram-negative antimicrobial prophylaxis reduces surgical site infections in hip arthroplasty. J Arthroplasty 2016;31:616–21.

29. Sewick A, Makani A, Wu C, et al. Does dual antibiotic prophylaxis better prevent surgical site infections in total joint arthroplasty? Clin Orthop Relat Res 2012;470:2702–7.

30. Illingworth KD, Mihalko WM, Parvizi J, et al. How to minimize infection and thereby maximize patient outcomes in total joint arthroplasty: a multicenter approach: AAOS exhibit selection. J Bone Joint Surg Am 2013;95:e50.

31. Campbell KA, Stein S, Looze C, et al. Antibiotic stewardship in orthopaedic surgery: principles and practice. J Am Acad Orthop Surg 2014;22:772–81.

32. Fishman N. Antimicrobial stewardship. Am J Infect Control 2006;34:S55–63 [discussion: S4–73].

33. Goff DA, Jankowski C, Tenover FC. Using rapid diagnostic tests to optimize antimicrobial selection in antimicrobial stewardship programs. Pharmacotherapy 2012;32:677–87.

34. Surgeons AAoO. The use of prophylactic antibiotics in orthopaedic medicine and the emergence of vancomycin-resistant bacteria. 1998. Revised 2002.

35. Meehan J, Jamali AA, Nguyen H. Prophylactic antibiotics in hip and knee arthroplasty. J Bone Joint Surg Am 2009;91:2480–90.

36. Smith EB, Wynne R, Joshi A, et al. Is it time to include vancomycin for routine perioperative antibiotic prophylaxis in total joint arthroplasty patients? J Arthroplasty 2012;27:55–60.

37. Iorio R, Osmani FA. Strategies to prevent periprosthetic joint infection after total knee arthroplasty and lessen the risk of readmission for the patient. J Am Acad Orthop Surg 2017;25(Suppl 1):S13–6.

38. Crowe B, Payne A, Evangelista PJ, et al. Risk factors for infection following total knee arthroplasty: a series of 3836 cases from one institution. J Arthroplasty 2015;30:2275–8.

39. Moucha CS, Clyburn T, Evans RP, et al. Modifiable risk factors for surgical site infection. J Bone Joint Surg Am 2011;93:398–404.

40. Cunningham DJ, Kavolus JJ 2nd, Bolognesi MP, et al. Common medical comorbidities correlated with poor outcomes in hip periprosthetic infection. J Arthroplasty 2017;32:241–5.e3.

41. Rezapoor M, Parvizi J. Prevention of periprosthetic joint infection. J Arthroplasty 2015;30:902–7.

42. Moucha CS, Clyburn T, Evans RP, et al. Modifiable risk factors for surgical site infection. J Bone Joint Surg Am 2011;93(4):398–404.

43. Alvi HM, Mednick RE, Krishnan V, et al. The effect of BMI on 30 day outcomes following total joint arthroplasty. J Arthroplasty 2015;30:1113–7.

44. Ravenscroft MJ, Harker J, Buch KA. A prospective, randomised, controlled trial comparing wound dressings used in hip and knee surgery: aquacel and tegaderm versus cutiplast. Ann R Coll Surg Engl 2006;88:18–22.

45. Duchman KR, Pugely AJ, Martin CT, et al. Operative time affects short-term complications in total joint arthroplasty. J Arthroplasty 2017;32:1285–91.

46. Namba RS, Paxton L, Fithian DC, et al. Obesity and perioperative morbidity in total hip and total knee arthroplasty patients. J Arthroplasty 2005;20:46–50.

47. Patel VP, Walsh M, Sehgal B, et al. Factors associated with prolonged wound drainage after primary total hip and knee arthroplasty. J Bone Joint Surg Am 2007;89:33–8.

48. Fehring TK, Odum SM, Griffin WL, et al. The obesity epidemic: its effect on total joint arthroplasty. J Arthroplasty 2007;22:71–6.

49. Schwarzkopf R, Lavery JA, Hooper J, et al. Bariatric surgery and time to total joint arthroplasty: does it affect readmission and complication rates? Obes Surg 2018;28:1395–401.

50. Singh JA, Lewallen DG. Diabetes: a risk factor for poor functional outcome after total knee arthroplasty. PLoS One 2013;8:e78991.

51. Cancienne JM, Werner BC, Browne JA. Is there a threshold value of hemoglobin a1c that predicts risk of infection following primary total hip arthroplasty? J Arthroplasty 2017;32:S236–40.

52. Yu S, Garvin KL, Healy WL, et al. Preventing hospital readmissions and limiting the complications associated with total joint arthroplasty. J Am Acad Orthop Surg 2015;23:e60–71.

53. Jamsen E, Nevalainen P, Eskelinen A, et al. Obesity, diabetes, and preoperative hyperglycemia as predictors of periprosthetic joint infection: a single-center analysis of 7181 primary hip and knee replacements for osteoarthritis. J Bone Joint Surg Am 2012;94:e101.

54. Iorio R, Williams KM, Marcantonio AJ, et al. Diabetes mellitus, hemoglobin A1C, and the incidence of total joint arthroplasty infection. J Arthroplasty 2012;27:726–729 e1.

55. Marchant MH Jr, Viens NA, Cook C, et al. The impact of glycemic control and diabetes mellitus on perioperative outcomes after total joint arthroplasty. J Bone Joint Surg Am 2009;91:1621–9.

56. Gupta S, Koirala J, Khardori R, et al. Infections in diabetes mellitus and hyperglycemia. Infect Dis Clin North Am 2007;21:617–38, vii.

57. Stryker LS. Modifying risk factors: strategies that work diabetes mellitus. J Arthroplasty 2016;31:1625–7.

58. Swensen S, Schwarzkopf R. Total joint arthroplasty in human immunodeficiency virus positive patients. Orthop Surg 2012;4:211–5.

59. Snir N, Wolfson TS, Schwarzkopf R, et al. Outcomes of total hip arthroplasty in human immunodeficiency virus-positive patients. J Arthroplasty 2014;29:157–61.

60. Morse CG, Mican JM, Jones EC, et al. The incidence and natural history of osteonecrosis in HIV-infected adults. Clin Infect Dis 2007;44:739–48.

61. Moller AM, Pedersen T, Villebro N, et al. Effect of smoking on early complications after elective orthopaedic surgery. J Bone Joint Surg Br 2003;85:178–81.

62. Duchman KR, Gao Y, Pugely AJ, et al. The effect of smoking on short-term complications following total hip and knee arthroplasty. J Bone Joint Surg Am 2015;97:1049–58.

63. Benowitz NL. Clinical pharmacology of nicotine. Annu Rev Med 1986;37:21–32.

64. Novikov DA, Swensen SJ, Buza JA 3rd, et al. The effect of smoking on ACL reconstruction: a systematic review. Phys Sportsmed 2016;44:335–41.

65. Singh JA, Schleck C, Harmsen WS, et al. Current tobacco use is associated with higher rates of implant revision and deep infection after total hip or knee arthroplasty: a prospective cohort study. BMC Med 2015;13:283.

66. Lindstrom D, Sadr Azodi O, Wladis A, et al. Effects of a perioperative smoking cessation intervention on postoperative complications: a randomized trial. Ann Surg 2008;248:739–45.

67. Moller AM, Villebro N, Pedersen T, et al. Effect of preoperative smoking intervention on postoperative complications: a randomised clinical trial. Lancet 2002;359:114–7.

68. Akhavan S, Nguyen LC, Chan V, et al. Impact of smoking cessation counseling prior to total joint arthroplasty. Orthopedics 2017;40:e323–8.

69. Blom AW, Brown J, Taylor AH, et al. Infection after total knee arthroplasty. J Bone Joint Surg Br 2004;86:688–91.

70. Brown NM, Cipriano CA, Moric M, et al. Dilute betadine lavage before closure for the prevention of acute postoperative deep periprosthetic joint infection. J Arthroplasty 2012;27:27–30.

71. von Keudell A, Canseco JA, Gomoll AH. Deleterious effects of diluted povidone-iodine on articular cartilage. J Arthroplasty 2013;28:918–21.

72. Frisch NB, Kadri OM, Tenbrunsel T, et al. Intraoperative chlorhexidine irrigation to prevent infection in

total hip and knee arthroplasty. Arthroplast Today 2017;3(4):294–7.

73. Smith TO, Sexton D, Mann C, et al. Sutures versus staples for skin closure in orthopaedic surgery: meta-analysis. BMJ 2010;340:c1199.

74. Livesey C, Wylde V, Descamps S, et al. Skin closure after total hip replacement: a randomised controlled trial of skin adhesive versus surgical staples. J Bone Joint Surg Br 2009;91:725–9.

75. Khan RJ, Fick D, Yao F, et al. A comparison of three methods of wound closure following arthroplasty: a prospective, randomised, controlled trial. J Bone Joint Surg Br 2006;88:238–42.

76. Campbell AL, Patrick DA Jr, Liabaud B, et al. Superficial wound closure complications with barbed sutures following knee arthroplasty. J Arthroplasty 2014;29:966–9.

77. Kim IOY, Anoushiravani AA, Long WJ, et al. A meta-analysis and systematic review evaluating skin closure after total knee arthroplasty-what is the best method? J Arthroplasty 2017;32:2920–7.

78. Krishnan R, MacNeil SD, Malvankar-Mehta MS. Comparing sutures versus staples for skin closure after orthopaedic surgery: systematic review and meta-analysis. BMJ Open 2016;6:e009257.

79. Gans I, Dormans JP, Spiegel DA, et al. Adjunctive vancomycin powder in pediatric spine surgery is safe. Spine 2013;38:1703–7.

80. Godil SS, Parker SL, O'Neill KR, et al. Comparative effectiveness and cost-benefit analysis of local application of vancomycin powder in posterior spinal fusion for spine trauma: clinical article. J Neurosurg Spine 2013;19:331–5.

81. Molinari RW, Khera OA, Molinari WJ 3rd. Prophylactic intraoperative powdered vancomycin and postoperative deep spinal wound infection: 1,512 consecutive surgical cases over a 6-year period. Eur Spine J 2012;21(Suppl 4):S476–82.

82. O'Neill KR, Smith JG, Abtahi AM, et al. Reduced surgical site infections in patients undergoing posterior spinal stabilization of traumatic injuries using vancomycin powder. Spine J 2011;11:641–6.

83. Schroeder JE, Girardi FP, Sandhu H, et al. The use of local vancomycin powder in degenerative spine surgery. Eur Spine J 2016;25:1029–33.

84. Wukich DK, Dikis JW, Monaco SJ, et al. Topically applied vancomycin powder reduces the rate of surgical site infection in diabetic patients undergoing foot and ankle surgery. Foot Ankle Int 2015;36: 1017–24.

85. Field FK, Kerstein MD. Overview of wound healing in a moist environment. Am J Surg 1994;167:2S–6S.

86. Vogt PM, Andree C, Breuing K, et al. Dry, moist, and wet skin wound repair. Ann Plast Surg 1995; 34:493–9 [discussion: 499–500].

87. Winter GD. Formation of the scab and the rate of epithelization of superficial wounds in the skin of the young domestic pig. Nature 1962;193:293–4.

88. Vasconcelos A, Cavaco-Paulo A. Wound dressings for a proteolytic-rich environment. Appl Microbiol Biotechnol 2011;90:445–60.

89. Grosso MJ, Berg A, LaRussa S, et al. Silver impregnated occlusive dressing reduces rates of acute periprosthetic joint infection after total joint arthroplasty. J Arthroplasty 2017;32(3).929–32.

90. Cai J, Karam JA, Parvizi J, et al. Aquacel surgical dressing reduces the rate of acute PJI following total joint arthroplasty: a case-control study. J Arthroplasty 2014;29:1098–100.

91. Dobbelaere A, Schuermans N, Smet S, et al. Comparative study of innovative postoperative wound dressings after total knee arthroplasty. Acta Orthop Belg 2015;81:454–61.

92. Ravnskog FA, Espehaug B, Indrekvam K. Randomised clinical trial comparing Hydrofiber and alginate dressings post-hip replacement. J Wound Care 2011;20:136–42.

93. Hopper GP, Deakin AH, Crane EO, et al. Enhancing patient recovery following lower limb arthroplasty with a modern wound dressing: a prospective, comparative audit. J Wound Care 2012;21:200–3.

94. Chowdhry M, Chen AF. Wound dressings for primary and revision total joint arthroplasty. Ann Transl Med 2015;3:268.

95. Williams C. An investigation of the benefits of Aquacel Hydrofibre wound dressing. Br J Nurs 1999;8:676–7, 680.

96. Dumville JC, Gray TA, Walter CJ, et al. Dressings for the prevention of surgical site infection. Cochrane Database Syst Rev 2014;(12):CD003091.

97. Ubbink DT, Vermeulen H, Goossens A, et al. Occlusive vs gauze dressings for local wound care in surgical patients: a randomized clinical trial. Arch Surg 2008;143:950–5.

Additive Manufacturing in Total Joint Arthroplasty

Sneha Prabha Narra, PhD[a],*, Peter N. Mittwede, MD[b], Sandra DeVincent Wolf, PhD[a], Kenneth L. Urish, MD, PhD[c,d]

KEYWORDS

- Additive manufacturing (AM) • 3-D printing • Electron beam melting (EBM)
- Laser powder bed fusion (LPBF) • Total joint arthroplasty • Orthopedics • Metal implants

---

KEY POINTS

- Additive manufacturing, popularly known as 3-D printing, is a layer-by-layer manufacturing process.
- Some of the advantages of additive manufacturing include using nonmachinable materials, fabricating complex geometries, and tailoring part properties.
- Currently available additive manufacturing processes, which fabricate parts with materials ranging from polymers to ceramics to metals, are discussed from the perspective of applicability in arthroplasty.
- Some applications of additive manufacturing in total joint arthroplasty include custom, patient-specific instrumentation and implants in hip and knee arthroplasty with new functionalities.
- There are gaps in additive manufacturing research, which, if addressed, have the potential to have a positive impact on the area of arthroplasty.

BACKGROUND

Hip and knee arthroplasty are common surgical procedures that have excellent long-term outcomes. The demand for these procedures continues to rise both in the United States and around the world.[1,2] With advancements in knowledge and technology, the implants used in total joint arthroplasty continue to undergo modifications to improve functional outcomes.[3,4] In recent years, there has been a growing interest in new manufacturing techniques that include custom implants and patient-specific instrumentation.[5,6] Although the literature is mixed on the outcomes of the early iterations of custom devices,[7] interest in them is unlikely to abate. In particular, additive manufacturing (AM) is a field that has been rapidly expanding in many industries and will likely play a major role in the future of total joint arthroplasty.

AM has become popular for producing lightweight and complex geometries (eg, hollow parts and cellular structures), offering an unparalleled level of design freedom, while also reducing material waste and the weight of components. This technology contrasts with traditional machining processes in which excess material is removed to produce the final part. This design flexibility makes AM attractive to the biomedical, aerospace, automotive, and energy sectors. For instance, General Electric

---

Disclosure Statement: None.

[a] NextManufacturing Center, College of Engineering, Carnegie Mellon University, 5000 Forbes Avenue, Pittsburgh, PA 15213, USA; [b] Department of Orthopaedic Surgery, University of Pittsburgh School of Medicine, 3471 Fifth Avenue, Suite 1010, Pittsburgh, PA 15213, USA; [c] Department of Orthopaedic Surgery, Arthritis and Arthroplasty Design Group, Magee-Womens Hospital, University of Pittsburgh School of Medicine, 300 Halket Street, Pittsburgh, PA 15213, USA; [d] The Bone and Joint Center, Magee-Womens Hospital, University of Pittsburgh School of Medicine, 300 Halket Street, Pittsburgh, PA 15213, USA

* Corresponding author.

E-mail address: snehaprabhanarra@gmail.com

invested in 2 major metal AM manufacturers—Arcam AB and Concept Laser GmbH—in 2016 to advance their AM business and research.[8] Given the current trends, investments in this technology are only expected to grow in the coming years.[9]

ADDITIVE MANUFACTURING BASICS

As the name suggests, AM is a process by which a final part is constructed by adding material successively in a layer-by-layer fashion, as shown in **Fig. 1**. A computer-aided design (CAD) model is first sliced into layers that are on the order of tens of microns and material is deposited into each layer successively, resulting in a complete part. This part is then postprocessed to result in a finished component. Current commercially available technologies can facilitate 3-D printing using a variety of materials, such as ceramics, composites, metals, plastics, and sand. Furthermore, active research is being conducted in the area of bioprinting to print cells, biomaterials, and biomolecules.[10]

From a classification standpoint, AM processes can be put into various categories depending on the materials (eg, polymers and metals) and the process used for fabrication. Polymers are widely used in different industries, primarily for prototyping purposes. Because the focus of this review is on arthroplasty applications, which primarily use metal alloy systems, metal AM is emphasized in this discussion. Metal AM can be further classified into nanoparticle jetting, binder jetting, powder bed fusion, and directed energy deposition processes.[11] The details of these processes and their applications in arthroplasty are discussed later.

Nanoparticle Jetting

In the nanoparticle jetting process, droplets containing the nanoparticles are first deposited onto the build-tray shown in **Fig. 2A**. Then, very high temperatures in the build envelope evaporate the liquid surrounding the nano-sized particles within a droplet, which brings the particles together. This process repeats at every layer, resulting in a final component, which then goes through a sintering process. The sintering process is performed to fuse the particles together, which fill any voids in the as-fabricated component. Nanoparticle jetting can be used to fabricate components with fine features and better surface finish compared with the processes that use larger powder sizes, such as powder bed fusion processes. XJet patented this technology and commercially manufactures the nanoparticle jetting machines.[12] This process can be used to additively manufacture both ceramic and metal parts. For example, medical materials such as zirconia can be used.

Binder Jetting

In the binder jetting process, liquid binder droplets are selectively deposited onto a powder bed within the boundaries described by the CAD model to bind the powder particles together, as shown in **Fig. 2B**.[13] This process is repeated for every layer in the part. At the end of the process, the part consists of powder particles that are held together by a binding agent. This is typically referred to as a "green part," which is then transferred to a curing oven to set the glue and further into a furnace for sintering and/or infiltration. During the sintering process, binder material evaporates and the powder particles sinter together, leaving the metal component behind. This results in shrinkage of approximately 30% to 40%. During the infiltration process, the

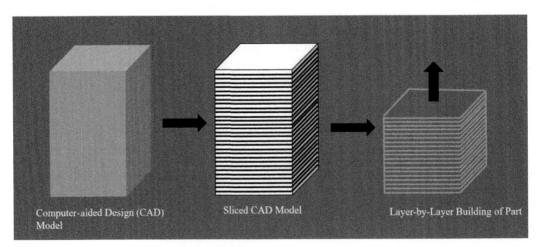

Computer-aided Design (CAD) Model   Sliced CAD Model   Layer-by-Layer Building of Part

Fig. 1. Layer-by-layer building of the component in AM.

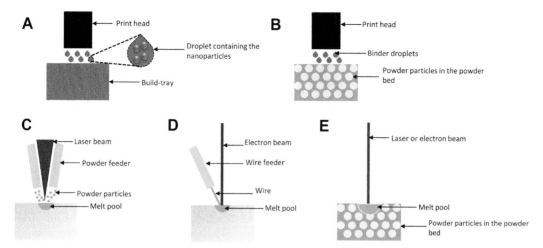

Fig. 2. Schematic of the metal AM processes: (*A*) nanoparticle jetting; (*B*) binder jetting; (*C*) Laser engineered net shaping; (*D*) electron beam wire feed; and (*E*) laser or electron beam powder bed fusion. (*Data from* Refs.[11,12,15,16])

bronze melts and is wicked into the part. On a comparative scale, infiltration results in less shrinkage (approximately 2%) than when just the sintering process is used. ExOne is the commercial manufacturer of the binder jetting machines to print components from metallic materials.[14] This process can be useful for prototyping and demonstration purposes in arthroplasty because it is cheaper than other metal AM processes.

Directed Energy Deposition

In the directed energy deposition process, the heat source is typically a laser or an electron beam. A traveling heat source is used to form a melt pool, and feedstock material is fed into the melt pool. This is similar to welding processes. Feedstock material can be in the form of powder or wire. Typically, when a laser beam is used as the heat source, the feedstock material is a powder. This powder is fed into the melt pool at every layer of the part during the deposition process as shown in **Fig. 2**C. This process is known as laser engineered net shaping (LENS).[15] Sandia National Laboratories developed this process and Optomec commercially manufactures LENS equipment. On the other hand, when the electron beam is the heat source, feedstock material is a metal wire, and this process is known as the electron beam wire feed (EBF3) process, as depicted in **Fig. 2**D.[16] National Aeronautics and Space Administration at Langley Research Center (Hampton, Virginia) developed this process and Sciaky commercially manufactures EBF3 equipment. EBF3 is a large-scale process suitable for medical equipment rather than implants. Materials, such as stainless steel and titanium, can be processed. On the other hand, LENS is

used for surface treatment of implants to improve their biocompatibility and performance.[17–19] It can also be used for fabrication of patient-specific implants and suitable for potential multimaterial applications and location-specific composition control of materials.[20,21] A variety of arthroplasty materials, such as stainless steel, titanium, and other composites, can be used for fabrication in the LENS process.

Powder Bed Fusion

This category of AM processes is widely used in both industrial production and research. In powder bed fusion processes, the feedstock material is a metal powder. Powder is spread onto a build plate, also known as a start plate, on which the parts are fabricated. At each layer, the powder is melted selectively as per the CAD model, using a laser or electron beam, followed by rapid solidification of the molten material. A schematic of this process is shown in **Fig. 2**E. The process of spreading the powder, melting, and solidification occurs at each layer until the part fabrication is complete. If a laser beam is used to melt the powder layer, the process is referred to as laser powder bed fusion (LPBF). If an electron beam is used to melt the powder layer, the process is known as electron beam melting (EBM). There are various companies commercializing the LPBF process (eg, EOS, SLM Solutions, Concept Laser GmbH, and TRUMPF). On the other hand, Arcam AB is currently the only commercial manufacturer of the EBM process. These processes can be used for various applications extending from prototyping to actual implants and medical devices. **Fig. 3** shows a Food and Drug Administration (FDA)–approved acetabular component with a rougher surface finish on the bone interface and smoother

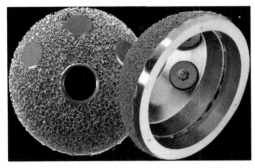

Fig. 3. Acetabular cup fabricated with Ti-6Al-4V using a LPBF process. (*left*) Rougher surface finish on the bone interface. (*right*) Smoother surface on the liner interface. (EOS M290 machine). (*Courtesy of* EOS North America; with permission.)

surface on the liner interface. Likewise, **Fig. 4** demonstrates the batch fabrication of knee implants using the EBM process. These illustrations demonstrate the applications of AM for patient-specific implants and for tailoring the part properties such as surface finish.

Various processes and related arthroplasty-specific applications are reviewed. To realize and further advance the full potential of any technology, however, it is important to understand the advantages and limitations of that technology. **Table 1** summarizes the major advantages and limitations of the state-of-the-art metal AM technologies.

APPLICATIONS IN TOTAL JOINT ARTHROPLASTY

According to the authors, the major current and potential applications of AM in arthroplasty can be divided into 3 main categories:

1. Patient-specific implants and instrumentation
2. Porous structures and functionally graded implants
3. Other novel applications

Because AM process-specific applications are discussed previously on different AM processes, the aim of this section is to summarize general applications of AM and their implications for total joint arthroplasty.

Patient-Specific Implants and Instrumentation
The concept of patient-specific instrumentation and implants has garnered much recent attention. The proposed potential benefits of patient-specific instrumentation in total knee arthroplasty include improving the accuracy of the bone cuts and thus the alignment of the implants and improving the operative time and efficiency (**Fig. 5**).[27] Although most studies thus far do not support any advantage of patient-specific instrumentation over conventional instrumentation,[7,28] improvements in the production and reliability of patient-specific instrumentation may increase their relevance and usefulness in the future, and AM technology could potentially provide this. AM has played a key role in the development of patient-specific implants in the field of craniomaxillofacial surgery and many researchers have explored this topic for different types of implants.[29–32] Although there are still only small case series that have reported the use of additively manufactured patient-specific implants in the field of arthroplasty,[33] there is much interest in this realm in the industrial sector, and surgeons will likely see an increased

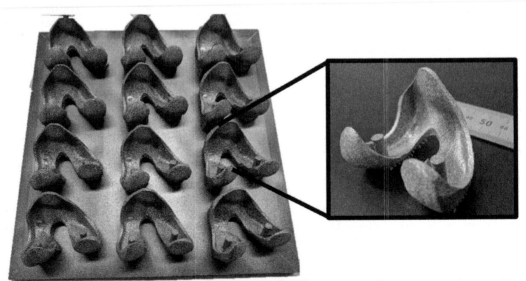

Fig. 4. Example of a knee implant prototype fabricated with Ti-6Al-4V using an EBM process (Arcam S12 machine). (*Courtesy of* NextManufacturing Center at Carnegie Mellon University, Pittsburgh, PA; with permission.)

Table 1
Advantages and limitations of state-of-the-art metal additive manufacturing processes in relation to total joint arthroplasty

Advantages	Limitations
• Allowing the fabrication of complex geometries that are otherwise not possible with traditional manufacturing methods for implants, such as porous mesh structures	• Machines and feedstock materials (if it is powder) are expensive[24] and may currently be cost prohibitive in arthroplasty.
• Enabling the fabrication of materials that are difficult to machine and are useful in arthroplasty, such as Ti-6Al-4V	• Standardization is challenging due to part-to-part and machine-to-machine variability,[25] which may be a barrier with regulatory agencies.
• Tailoring the microstructure and properties based on individual patient needs, such as adjusting the density of the implant to match with bone density[22]	• Producing uniform microstructure and defect-free parts is a work in progress, which might require additional postprocessing that adds to the cost of the implant.
• Enabling the fabrication of lightweight parts that results in reduced material waste, such as hollow structures	• Successful fabrication of parts with new materials and design involves extensive experimentation, which is expensive and time consuming, and limits the utilization of the full potential of the technology.[26]
• Enabling the consolidation of components to reduce the assembly time and create new design opportunities[23]	• Postprocessing costs also contribute to the total fabrication costs, which can make the process expensive for applications, such as bearing surfaces, that require a smooth surface finish.

use for this technology moving forward. In particular, complex revision hip arthroplasty cases are an area where AM technology could be applied in the current environment but these applications will likely expand as the characteristics and potential benefits of additively manufactured constructs become better understood.[34]

Porous Structures and Functionally Graded Implants

The layer-by-layer nature of AM makes it popular for fabricating complex geometries. This has proved especially advantageous for medical implants. **Fig. 6** shows the possibility of fabricating fine mesh structures and the ability to tailor mesh structures to change the density and resulting stiffness of the fabricated part.[35] Murr and colleagues[22] demonstrated the concepts

of variable density and stiffness in total knee and total hip implants using Ti-6Al-4V and Co-29Cr-6Mo via the EBM process. For instance, the inner surface of the Co-29Cr-6Mo femoral knee implant and outer surface of the Ti-6Al-4V acetabular cup are made porous to improve bone ingrowth and to modify the stiffness to address stress shielding. Arabnejad and

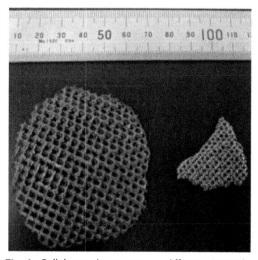

Fig. 6. Cellular mesh structures at different size scales fabricated with Ti-6Al-4V using an EBM process (Arcam S12 machine). Different meshes result in different part densities and mechanical properties. (*Courtesy of* NextManufacturing Center at Carnegie Mellon University, Pittsburgh, PA; with permission.)

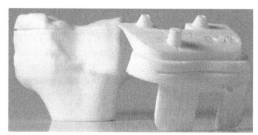

Fig. 5. Nylon 12 EOS PA2200 patient-specific cutting guide fabricated using an LPBF process (EOS P396 machine). (*Courtesy of* EOS North America; with permission.)

colleagues implemented the tailoring of mesh structures to generate a functionally-graded femoral stem that has an optimum relative density distribution. In vitro tests revealed substantial reduction in stress shielding illustrating that tailoring densities and stiffness were critical for minimizing the stress shielding effects.[36] For cementless orthopedic implants, Harrison and colleagues[37] demonstrated that AM can be used to fabricate novel surface architectures to replace traditional surface coatings. In this study, hip stem components with OsteoAnchor surface architecture made out of Ti-6Al-4V were compared with the hip stems with standard plasma sprayed titanium coatings that are implanted in animals. Results suggested that the OsetoAnchor surface achieved with AM had superior primary fixation and better bone in-growth. This work suggests that AM can be used as a tool to fabricate and test customized surface architectures. Interested readers may want to review the vast literature on the impact of porous structures and functionally graded implants on the stability and the life of an implant.

Novel Applications

The layer-by-layer manufacturing of materials and the ability to fabricate with a variety of materials and geometries opens up opportunities to pursue new research. For instance, use of AM has been suggested as an alternative to the current procedures to treat periprosthetic infections.[38] Kim and colleagues[38] proposed using AM to print polylactic acid liners, which can either have antibiotics embedded into them or consist of reservoirs and microchannels for controlled drug delivery. Similarly, Bezuidenhout and colleagues[39] suggested the possibility of using AM for drug delivery. In the same work, challenges related to the development of such implants are discussed, highlighting the need for collaboration among stakeholders to realize these novel applications. For in situ measurements of implant performance, Micolini and colleagues[40] demonstrated the use of AM to fabricate a polymer sensor array with conductive polyaniline that can be embedded into implants for in-situ measurement of load transmission. Besides that, AM is also being used as a prototyping tool for testing new research approaches. As an example, Uklejewski and colleagues[41] used selective laser melting to fabricate a biomimetic multispiked connecting scaffold in their efforts to develop noncemented stemless resurfacing hip arthroplasty endoprostheses. These examples demonstrate that AM holds potential to revolutionize the state-of-the-art in the implant industry and catalyze the industry toward improving health care.

CHALLENGES AND OPPORTUNITIES FOR FUTURE RESEARCH

AM applications in arthroplasty include prototyping, actual functional implants, and many potential novel applications that are otherwise not viable through traditional manufacturing. Although this sounds promising, there are challenges associated with the technology that are hindering its widespread adoption. From the authors' perspective, the push for using AM has to be led by the surgeons and, more specifically, through their interest in customizable implants. Currently, due to the high costs of AM, this technology is mainly limited to usage for revision arthroplasty procedures. Reducing the cost of AM can potentially lead to a more widespread adoption of AM techniques beyond just revisions. Another practical challenge is the process of obtaining approval from the FDA, which can be extensive and cumbersome. Recently, the FDA issued technical considerations for additively manufactured devices to serve as a guide for industry as well as for FDA staff who are considering to use AM.[42] Unlike for some of the established manufacturing practices, such as machining and casting, it is reasonable to say that for a new technology like AM, the burden of proof is higher.

The opportunities for future research lie in addressing these challenges. To address the higher costs of using AM, Laureijs and colleagues[24] concluded that reducing the cost associated with feedstock material can reduce the manufacturing costs of the implants. One way to accomplish this is to develop methods to use inexpensive feedstock materials that can provide comparable performance to the current feedstock material. Additionally, cost can be reduced by minimizing the scrap material from the fabricated parts. Typically, scrap includes support structures and extra material added to the component to achieve tolerances after machining. Furthermore, cost can also be reduced by increasing the reuse of materials. For FDA approval purposes, standards can be developed by understanding the properties of the fabricated components and the effect of processing conditions on the part properties. It is also important to understand and control the process variability and this can be done by implementing in situ monitoring and controls.[25,43] To encourage surgeons to use AM, new functionalities should be explored and incorporated into the additively manufactured implants and devices. Specifically, the advantages offered by AM, such as geometric freedom and location-specific control of properties, should be leveraged to address the challenges faced by surgeons. In conclusion, this review highlights the potential of AM to revolutionize the area of total joint arthroplasty and research opportunities that lie at the intersection of addressing the current challenges in AM and developing innovative approaches in arthroplasty.

ACKNOWLEDGMENTS

Dr S.P. Narra is supported by the NextManufacturing Center at Carnegie Mellon University. Dr K.L. Urish is supported in part by the National Institute of Arthritis and Musculoskeletal and Skin Diseases (NIAMS K08AR071494), the National Center for Advancing Translational Sciences (NCATS KL2TR0001856), and the Orthopaedic Research and Education Foundation. The authors thank EOS North America for providing the images of the acetabular cup and patient-specific cutting guide. The authors would also like to thank graduate students Joseph Pauza, Ali Alp Gurer, Vignesh Viswanathan, Mahemaa Rajasekaran, Daming Ding, and Yumin Yan at Carnegie Mellon University for generously offering us images of the knee implant prototype used in this article. The authors would like to acknowledge the NextManufacturing Center at Carnegie Mellon University for providing the images of the components fabricated on the Arcam S12.

REFERENCES

1. Kurtz SM, Ong KL, Lau E, et al. Impact of the economic downturn on total joint replacement demand in the United States: updated projections to 2021. J Bone Joint Surg Am 2014;96(8):624–30.
2. Inacio MCS, Graves SE, Pratt NL, et al. Increase in total joint arthroplasty projected from 2014 to 2046 in Australia: a conservative local model with international implications. Clin Orthop Relat Res 2017;475(8):2130–7.
3. Lachiewicz PF, Kleeman LT, Seyler T. Bearing surfaces for total hip arthroplasty. J Am Acad Orthop Surg 2018;26(2):45–57.
4. Nieuwenhuijse MJ, Nelissen RGHH, Schoones JW, et al. Appraisal of evidence base for introduction of new implants in hip and knee replacement: a Systematic review of five widely used device technologies. BMJ 2014;349:g5133.
5. Nguyen LCL, Lehil MS, Bozic KJ. Trends in total knee arthroplasty implant utilization. J Arthroplasty 2015;30(5):739–42.
6. Berend ME, Berend KR, Lombardi AV, et al. The patient-specific Triflange acetabular implant for revision total hip arthroplasty in patients with severe acetabular defects: planning, implantation, and results. Bone Joint J 2018;100B(1):50–4.
7. Sassoon A, Nam D, Nunley R, et al. Systematic review of patient-specific instrumentation in total knee arthroplasty: new but not improved. Clin Orthop Relat Res 2015;473(1):151–8.
8. GE makes significant progress with investments in additive equipment companies | GE Additive. Available at: https://www.ge.com/additive/press-releases/ge-makes-significant-progress-investments-additive-equipment-companies. Accessed July 1, 2018.
9. 3D Printing Industry to 2027 | Market Reports | Smithers Pira. Smithers Pira. Available at: https://www.smitherspira.com/industry-market-reports/printing/the-future-of-3d-printing-to-2027. Accessed May 17, 2018.
10. Seol YJ, Kang HW, Lee SJ, et al. Bioprinting technology and its applications. Eur J Cardiothorac Surg 2014;46(3):342–8.
11. 3D HUBS. What is 3D Printing? The definitive guide to additive manufacturing. 3Dhubs.Com. 2017. Available at: https://www.3dhubs.com/what-is-3d-printing. Accessed March 3, 2017.
12. XJet. X-Jet technology. Available at: http://www.xjet3d.com/technology.html. Accessed March 3, 2017.
13. Sachs E, Cima M, Williams P, et al. Three dimensional printing: rapid tooling and prototypes directly from a CAD model. J Eng Ind 1992;114:481–8.
14. What Is Binder Jetting? | ExOne. 2016. Available at: http://www.exone.com/Resources/Technology-Overview/What-is-Binder-Jetting. Accessed March 3, 2017.
15. Griffith M, Keicher D. Free form fabrication of metallic components using laser engineered net shaping (LENS). In: Solid Freeform Fabrication Proceedings. Austin (TX); 1996:125–32.
16. Taminger K, Hafley R. Electron beam freeform fabrication: a rapid metal deposition process. In: Proceedings of the 3rd Annual Automotive Composites Conference. Troy; 2003:9–10. Available at: https://ntrs.nasa.gov/archive/nasa/casi.ntrs.nasa.gov/20040042496.pdf. Accessed March 3, 2017.
17. Emmelmann C, Scheinemann P, Munsch M, et al. Laser additive manufacturing of modified implant surfaces with osseointegrative characteristics. Phys Procedia 2011;12:375–84.
18. Janaki Ram G, Yang Y, Stucker BE. Deposition of Ti/TiC composite coatings on implant structures using laser engineered net shaping. In: Proceedings of Solid Freeform Fabrication Symposium. Austin (TX); 2007:527–39.
19. Roy M, Bandyopadhyay A, Bose S. In vitro antimicrobial and biological properties of laser assisted tricalcium phosphate coating on titanium for load bearing implant. Mater Sci Eng C 2009;29(6):1965–8.

20. Vamsi Krishna B, Xue W, Bose S, et al. Engineered porous metals for implants. JOM 2008;60(5):45–8.

21. Das M, Balla VK, Kumar TSS, et al. Fabrication of biomedical implants using laser engineered net shaping (LENS™). Trans Indian Ceram Soc 2013; 72(3):169–74.

22. Murr LE, Gaytan SM, Martinez E, et al. Next generation orthopaedic implants by additive manufacturing using electron beam melting. Int J Biomater 2012; 2012:245727.

23. Schmelzle J, Kline EV, Dickman CJ, et al. (Re) Designing for part consolidation: understanding the challenges of metal additive manufacturing. J Mech Des 2015;137(11):111404.

24. Laureijs RE, Roca JB, Narra SP, et al. Metal additive manufacturing: cost competitive beyond low volumes. J Manuf Sci Eng Trans ASME 2017; 139(8).

25. Herderick E. Additive manufacturing of metals: a review. Columbus (OH): Materials Science and Technology (MS&T); 2011. p. 1413–25.

26. Beuth J, Fox J, Gockel J, et al. Process mapping for qualification across multiple direct metal additive manufacturing processes. In: Proceedings of Solid Freeform Fabrication Symposium. Austin (TX); 2013:655–5.

27. Urish KL, Conditt M, Roche M, et al. Robotic total knee arthroplasty: surgical assistant for a customized normal kinematic knee. Orthopedics 2016; 39(5):e822–7.

28. Thienpont E, Schwab PE, Fennema P. A systematic review and meta-analysis of patient-specific instrumentation for improving alignment of the components in total knee replacement. Bone Joint J 2014;96 B(8):1052–61.

29. Nickels L. World's first patient-specific jaw implant. Metal Powder Report 2012;67(2):12–4.

30. Jardini AL, Larosa MA, Filho RM, et al. Cranial reconstruction: 3D biomodel and custom-built implant created using additive manufacturing. J Craniomaxillofac Surg 2014;42(8):1877–84.

31. Dérand P, Rännar L-E, Hirsch J-M. Imaging, virtual planning, design, and production of patient-specific implants and clinical validation in craniomaxillofacial surgery. Craniomaxillofac Trauma Reconstr 2012;05(03):137–44.

32. Salmi M, Tuomi J, Paloheimo K, et al. Patient-specific reconstruction with 3D modeling and DMLS additive manufacturing. Rapid Prototyp J 2012; 18(3):209–14.

33. Colen S, Harake R, De Haan J, et al. A modified custom-made triflanged acetabular reconstruction ring (MCTARR) for revision hip arthroplasty with severe acetabular defects. Acta Orthop Belg 2013;79(1):71–5. Available at: http://www.ncbi.nlm.nih.gov/pubmed/23547519. Accessed June 9, 2018.

34. Cheng A, Humayun A, Cohen DJ, et al. Additively manufactured 3D porous Ti-6Al-4V constructs mimic trabecular bone structure and regulate osteoblast proliferation, differentiation and local factor production in a porosity and surface roughness dependent manner. Biofabrication 2014;6(4):045007.

35. Gibson LJ, Ashby MF. Cellular solids. Cambridge (UK): Cambridge University Press; 1997. https://doi.org/10.1017/CBO9781139878326

36. Arabnejad S, Johnston B, Tanzer M, et al. Fully porous 3D printed titanium femoral stem to reduce stress-shielding following total hip arthroplasty. J Orthop Res 2017;35(8):1774–83.

37. Harrison N, Field JR, Quondamatteo F, et al. Preclinical trial of a novel surface architecture for improved primary fixation of cementless orthopaedic implants. Clin Biomech 2014;29(8):861–8.

38. Kim TWB, Lopez OJ, Sharkey JP, et al. 3D printed liner for treatment of periprosthetic joint infections. Med Hypotheses 2017;102:65–8.

39. Bezuidenhout MB, Dimitrov DM, Van Staden AD, et al. Titanium-based hip stems with drug delivery functionality through additive manufacturing. Biomed Res Int 2015;2015:1–11.

40. Micolini C, Holness F, Johnson J, et al. Assessment of embedded conjugated polymer sensor arrays for potential load transmission measurement in orthopaedic implants. Sensors (Basel) 2017;17(12):2768.

41. Uklejewski R, Rogala P, Winiecki M, et al. Preliminary results of implantation in animal model and osteoblast culture evaluation of prototypes of biomimetic multispiked connecting scaffold for noncemented stemless resurfacing hip arthroplasty endoprostheses. Biomed Res Int 2013; 2013:689089.

42. FDA. Technical Considerations for Additive Manufactured Medical Devices - Guidance for Industry and Food and Drug Administration Staff.; 2017. Available at: https://www.fda.gov/downloads/MedicalDevices/DeviceRegulationandGuidance/GuidanceDocuments/UCM499809.pdf. Accessed May 16, 2018.

43. Frazier WE. Metal additive manufacturing: a review. J Mater Eng Perform 2014;23(6):1917–28.

Nanopatterning and Bioprinting in Orthopedic Surgery

Felasfa M. Wodajo, MD[a,b,c,*], Adam E. Jakus, PhD[d]

KEYWORDS

- Periprosthetic infection • Nanopatterning • Biofilm • Iodine-coated orthopedic implants
- Bioprinting • Tissue fabrication • Tissue regeneration • Advanced biomaterials

KEY POINTS

- Metal surface roughness and chemistry at the nanoscale affect bacterial adhesion.
- Nanoscale pillars, mimicking those found on insect wings, inhibit bacterial growth in vitro.
- Titanium implants anodized with iodine demonstrate promising preliminary resistance to infection.
- Similarities and differences between traditional medical 3D printing and cell and tissue 3D printing and materials for tissue regeneration are explored in this article.
- Bioprinting processes, requirements, cell selection, and sourcing are introduced in this article.

PART 1: ANTIMICROBIAL NANOPATTERNING AND SURFACE MODIFICATIONS IN ORTHOPEDIC SURGERY

Introduction

Additive manufacturing (3-dimensional or "3D printing") has opened the door for more sophisticated orthopedic implants. However, regardless of design architecture, bacterial infection of musculoskeletal implants will remains a major mode of failure, often at great cost and morbidity to the patient. Catastrophic orthopedic infections are often due to otherwise indolent organisms, such as *Staphylococcus epidermidis*, due to the ability of these bacteria to form a protein and polysaccharide-rich biofilm. This biofilm protects the bacteria from the effects of antimicrobial agents and thus condemns the patient to further surgery, sometimes multiple, to remove and replace the implant.

Although surgeons may equate the presence of periprosthetic infection with an automatic need for explantation surgery, the real culprit is the biofilm. For example, periprosthetic infections due to *Mycobacterium tuberculosis*, which does not produce significant biofilm, can be successfully treated without removal of the affected implant.[1]

Bacteria have evolved a range of adhesive proteins for attachment to various surfaces. From the attachment of bacteria to a metal surface to formation of this biofilm is a rapid and efficient process, often completed within 12 to 18 hours of contact between bacteria and the host surface. Many techniques have been attempted to modify implant surfaces in order

No pertinent conflicts; full disclosures at http://www7.aaos.org/Education/disclosure/search.aspx.
Disclosure Statement: A.E. Jakus is a co-founder and shareholder in Dimension Inx, LLC, which designs, develops, manufactures, and sells new 3D-printable materials and end-use products for medical and nonmedical applications. A.E. Jakus is currently full-time Chief Technology Officer of Dimension Inx, LLC.
[a] Virginia Cancer Specialists, 8503 Arlington Boulevard, Suite 400, Fairfax, VA 22031, USA; [b] Orthopedic Surgery, VCU School of Medicine, Inova Campus, Fairfax, VA 22042, USA; [c] Orthopedic Surgery, Georgetown University Hospital, Washington, DC 20007, USA; [d] Dimension Inx LLC, 303 East Superior Street, 11th Floor, Chicago, IL 60611, USA
* Corresponding author. Virginia Cancer Specialists, 8503 Arlington Boulevard, Suite 400, Fairfax, VA 22031.
E-mail address: wodajo@sarcoma.md

to reduce the risk of infection. These techniques can be broadly grouped into the following three categories:

1. Passive surfaces which do not release bactericidal agents;
2. Active surfaces with preincorporated bactericidal agents;
3. Antibacterial carriers or coatings applied at surgery[2]

Of these, categories 2 and 3 have the most clinical data thus far. In particular, implants with surfaces that release metal ions such as silver and iodine that have bactericidal properties are already in use in Europe and Japan, respectively. Incorporating antibiotics onto implant surfaces, although intuitively attractive, will likely have an uphill course in gaining US regulatory approval, in large part because of concerns about creating resistant bacterial species.[2,3] However, natural occurring peptides with antibacterial properties may be a future alternative to antibiotics.[5]

Passive surfaces that inhibit bacterial growth have thus far been seen in preclinical work but show some promising results. These surfaces have features measured in nanometers and thus are not "printed" in same way as 3D printing. Rather, they are etched with electron beams, by chemical processes, or by using specialized lithography processes. These techniques are discussed later.

Passive Surfaces and Nanopatterning

The observation that insect wings possess an antimicrobial capacity based purely on their biophysical characteristics opened a venue for investigations on whether an analogous function could be imparted to implanted biomaterials. The initial observations were made on cicada wings, which demonstrated an ability to inhibit growth of gram-negative organisms, such as *Pseudomonas aeruginosa*. Electron microscopy has demonstrated these wings to be covered by "nanopillars," arranged spaced 170 nm apart and each ~200 nm tall (Fig. 1).[6]

It is important to realize that, although large-scale production of surface details at the micron level are routine in the electronics industry, fine detail features at the nanometer scale are not achievable with the wavelengths of light used in typical wafer production. Resolutions obtained in microfabrication laboratories today decrease in size to 100 nm. Use of deep UV light allows the fabrication of features of sizes in decreasing size to 50 nm. However, masks can also be made using techniques other than light

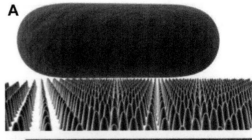
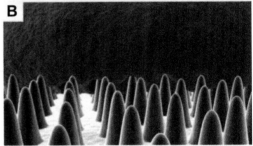
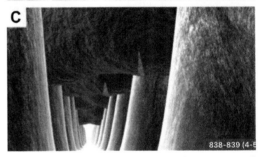

838-839 (4-5

Fig. 1. Biophysical model of the cicada wing nanopillars and bacterial cells. (A) Bacteria come into contact and (B) adsorb onto the nanopillars causing (C) the outer layer to rupture. (*From* Pogodin S, Hasan J, Baulin VA, et al. Biophysical model of bacterial cell interactions with nanopatterned cicada wing surfaces. Biophys J 2013;104(4):838; with permission.)

such as "dry etching," "nanoimprint lithography," which involves the use of polymers and colloids to generate a 2-dimensional (2D) structure. Surface chemical treatments can also be used to create nanotopographies that are random but with uniform roughness. More precise is electron beam lithography, in which an electron beam is used to etch a surface similarly to photolithography. By using this technique, resolutions as low as 15 nm can be achieved, but the process is usually slow and thus costly. In general, the technical challenge in producing surface features at the nanoscale level, produced over large areas, is a significant impediment in terms of cost and time at this time.[7]

Attachment between cells and surfaces is mediated by multiple proteins, the most common being the integrin family. Upon adhesion to a substrate, cells probe the environment with nanometer scale filopodia. More stable adhesions result in less retraction of filopodia. As these processes attach, they serve as anchor points for net movement via lamellipodia. By modulating the stability of these anchor points, nanoscale features can direct net movement of cells (Fig. 2).[7]

In addition to effects on cell movement, nanoscale topography appears to have differential effects based on cell type or even stimulate cell differentiation selectively. In one experiment, nanoscale pits were formed with electron beam lithography on polymethyl methacrylate (PMMA) in random, hexagonal, and square arrangements. When human mesenchymal stem cells were cultured on these surfaces, it was noted that surfaces with square arrangement and average displacement between pits of 20 nm or 50 nm were more likely, compared with other distances, to promote growth of cells positive for osteocalcin and osteopontin, markers of osteoblast differentiation.[7]

Surface chemistry of a biomaterial can also play a significant role in the ability of bacteria to adhere and multiply. In a series of experiments, one group demonstrated a dramatic reduction in the ability of sulfate-reducing bacteria to adhere to steel. These bacteria are major contributors to corrosion of oil and gas pipelines. The group tested anodization of steel in a NaOH solution at various voltages. As expected, the steel's surface roughness and "water contact angle," a measure of hydrophobicity, varied depending on the anodization voltage. They found that the maximum hydrophobicity, as indicated by the largest contact angle, was achieved at at 2.0 V. Compared with bare steel, the surface

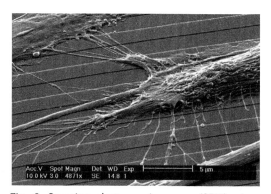

Fig. 2. Scanning electron microscope (SEM) micrograph of eukaryotic cells elongating longitudinally along nanoscale grooves while filopodia probe randomly. (From Anselme K, Davidson P, Popa AM, et al. The interaction of cells and bacteria with surfaces structured at the nanometre scale. Acta Biomater 2010;6(10):3830; with permission.)

produced using this relatively simple, one-step technique demonstrated a 23.5-fold reduction of bacterial adhesion.[8]

In addition to the above effects, an important factor in bacterial adhesion is the interplay between proteins present in the biological media and bacteria. When biomaterial surfaces interact with biological systems, whether in vitro or in vivo, they are immediately coated by native proteins. One reason titanium demonstrates excellent biocompatibility is due to the incorporation of a surface layer of inert titanium oxide. To test the interaction between proteins and bacterial adhesion, one group produced a series of titania with carefully regulated nanoscale morphology of this titanium oxide layer. They found that protein adsorption increases with surface roughness. Bacterial adhesion also initially increased with surface roughness. However, they observed a significant decrease of bacterial biofilm formation and adhesion with the further increase of roughness. From these findings, they proposed that a thick layer of adsorbed protein may reduce bacterial growth by directly interfering with adhesion as well as by flattening the nanoscale surface.[9]

Finally, Dickson and colleagues[10] fabricated a simulation of the nanopillars seen on cicada wings using silicon molds using several techniques, including silicone imprint molds of cicada wings. The nanopillars were fabricated on PMMA at varying periodicities, and the samples were cultured with Escherichia coli. Scanning electron micrographs of the tested film samples are seen in Fig. 3. The group found that films with nanopillars had a higher percentage of dead bacteria than the flat ones, with smaller and more closely spaced pillars more effective than wider spaced pillars (Fig. 4). In addition, the investigators noted that the pillars had a bactericidal action, beyond the theoretic inhibition of adhesion, as bacterial load in the overlying aqueous suspension decreased by 50% over 24 hours.

Active Antibacterial Surfaces
Preincorporated antibacterial surfaces provide simplicity for the surgeon, but in the United States likely involve the need for Food and Drug Administration (FDA) clearance. Nevertheless, there are several promising avenues that take advantage of biologic and non-biologic agents.

Biologic agents
Precoating metallic surfaces with endogenous proteins, such as albumin, fibronectin, fibrinogen, or some lipids, has been proposed to promote rapid adhesion by eukaryotic cells. The

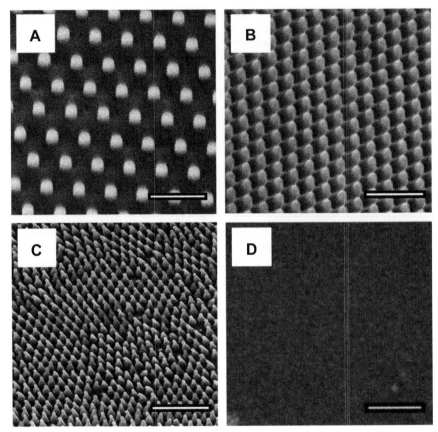

Fig. 3. SEM micrographs of PMMA with nanopillars at various periodicities: (*A*) 600 nm, (*B*) 300 nm, (*C*) 200 nm replicate of cicada wing, and (*D*) flat control. Scale bars, 1 μm. (*From* Dickson MN, Liang EI, Rodriguez LA, et al. Nanopatterned polymer surfaces with bactericidal properties. Biointerphases 2015;10(2):021010; with permission.)

concept underlying this proposal is one given the name "race for the surface" popularized by Gristina and colleagues[3,4] in 1988 wherein the risk of biomaterial bacterial infection can be reduced if mammalian cell adhesion blocks bacterial adhesion.

A large number of naturally occurring peptides have been investigated that have antimicrobial characteristics. These proteins are collectively termed host defense peptides (HDPs) and currently number more than 1000. HDPs are part of the innate immune system and act as a first line of defense against infection. Classification of the major HDP families in mammals has thus far been by their protein structure, for example, defensins, cathelicidins, and histatins. However, newer information is widening the complexity of the roles these peptides play within the immune system and may lead to modification of these classifications. For example, proteins that were previously thought to be chemo-attractants are now understood to orchestrate an antimicrobial role. Other

proteins have more direct microbicidal and others immunomodulatory roles.[5]

Despite, or perhaps due to, the breadth of the HDP family, attempts at clinical applications have not yet yielded definitive results. Systemic application of HDPs has been hampered by significant toxicity. However, topical application may hold more promise. Polymyxin-containing topical ointments are commercially available. Intranasal delivery of HDP in an animal model of *Pseudomonas aeurignosa* pneumonia resulted in eradicating biofilm and reducing colony-forming units in nasal effluent.[5]

One group modified a previously described HDP and tested it in a model of *Candida albicans* biofilm infection. They modified an existing peptide, LL-37, which is known to diminish the attachment of bacterial cells and downregulate genes for biofilm development in multiple gram-positive and gram-negative bacteria. The group found their derived peptide worked synergistically with antifungal antibiotics to inhibit the formation of *C albicans* biofilm on titanium

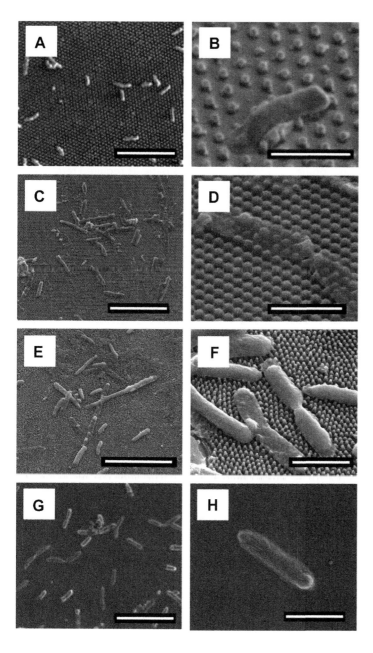

Fig. 4. SEM micrographs of bacteria on patterned PMMA surfaces of varying periodicities: (*A, B*) 600 nm, (*C, D*) 300 nm, (*E, F*) P200 nm, and (*G, H*) flat control. (*B*) Note how bacteria deflate as they drape across several pillars with evidence of leakage of cytoplasm. Scale bars, 10 μm on left, 2 μm on right. (*From* Dickson MN, Liang EI, Rodriguez LA, et al. Nanopatterned polymer surfaces with bactericidal properties. Biointerphases 2015;10(2):021010; with permission.)

disks and polystyrene pegs. It also reduced the number of *S epidermidis* bacteria when tested with mixed flora. Although fungal infections constitute less than 1% of orthopedic joint prosthesis infections,[11] the investigators note that coinfection of *C albicans* and *S epidermidis* is an important problem in neonatal intensive care units where it is associated with increased mortality compared with single-species infections. Importantly, the peptide was not found to be toxic for human osteoblasts, mesenchymal stromal cells, and endothelial cells.[12]

Non-biologic agents

Animal studies have demonstrated decreased infection rates of metal implants coated with antibiotic-containing hydroxyapatite, and in vitro studies have demonstrated resistance to infection of metal devices coated with chlorhexidine-loaded hydroxyapatite.[2]

Antimicrobial metals have a longer history of use in implants. Silver was the preferred material for indwelling catheters in gynecology as early as in the middle of the nineteenth century.[11] However, although the antimicrobial effects of silver have long been established, its use in permanent implants has raised concerns about potential toxicity of accumulated silver ions.[12]

More recent work from Japan has demonstrated clinical efficacy of iodine-coated orthopedic implants. In this instance, the group took advantage of the natural oxide that coats titanium implants and that promotes its excellent biocompatibility. Using povidone-iodine as the electrolyte during anodization, iodine can be trapped in the oxide layer in nanoscale pores (Fig. 5).[13] The antimicrobial action of iodine functions by denaturing proteins. The investigators had previously demonstrated that fibroblast proliferation and osseointegration in a rabbit model were unaffected by the presence of this iodine coating. The antibacterial spectrum of iodine is very broad, including not only bacteria but also viruses, tubercle bacilli, and fungi. Iodine does not cause drug resistance as would be induced by the administration of antibiotics. Moreover, iodine is a component of the thyroid hormone and is excreted by the kidneys.[14]

Iodine-supported implants were tested in vitro using titanium disks cultured with *Staphylococcus aureus* as well as in rats with percutaneously implanted Kirschner wires. In both cases, the rate of biofilm formation was markedly lower in iodine-supported implants compared with controls.[15]

More impressive were clinical results demonstrated by the group. In 158 patients without preexisting infection treated with iodine-supported implants that included a mix of external fixators, spinal and joint implants, there were 3 infections for a very low infection rate of 1.9%. One of these patients required removal of Marlex mesh, whereas the other 2 were cured with intravenous antibiotics only. Another 66 patients with prosthetic joint infections were treated with one- and 2-stage revisions using iodine-supported implants (Fig. 6). At a mean follow-up of 18.4 months, only one patient developed what the investigators termed "late hematogenous infection" 2 years after revision surgery, and one had a suspected iodine allergy. There were no signs of infection in the rest of the cohort at last follow-up.[14]

Intraoperatively Applied Coatings

The use of biocompatible or resorbable antibiotic carriers is not new to orthopedics. The most widely used intraoperatively modified coating is antibiotic-loaded methyl methacrylate. Long-term arthroplasty registry studies comparing the use of cement with and without antibiotics have shown that revision rates due to infection were lower with use of antibiotic-containing cement. Interestingly, revisions for aseptic loosening were also less frequent, suggesting the possibility that some cases of aseptic loosening were in fact due to undetected organisms.[16] It is relevant to recall that the bulk of antibiotic from methyl methacrylate is released within 4 weeks.[17] Thus, the long-term benefit of antibiotic-containing cement may well be to inhibition of initial biofilm formation.

However, methyl methacrylate was not designed as an antibiotic carrier, and in vitro studies where bacteria are introduced to antibiotic-loaded cement have shown that bacterial microcolonies persist within the surface that could potentially represent resistant "small" colonies.[18]

In an attempt to overcome the disadvantages of methyl methacrylate, one group performed in vitro testing of a fast-resorbing hydrogel loaded with antibiotic (Fig. 7). Rapid release of the antibiotic could prevent the potential problem of antimicrobial resistance. Use of a temporary coating could also avoid blocking osteointegration, as would happen with a permanent coating. Using a hydrogel rather than

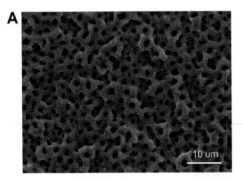

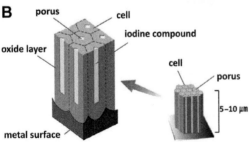

Fig. 5. Electron micrograph of the oxide layer: (A) more than 50,000 pores/mm². (B) Diagram of the anodizing porous membrane. (From Tsuchiya H, Shirai T, Nishida H, et al. Innovative antimicrobial coating of titanium implants with iodine. J Orthop Sci 2012;17(5):596; with permission.)

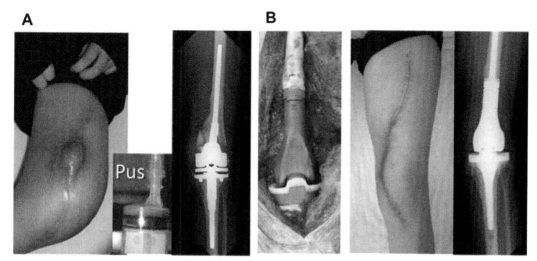

Fig. 6. (A) Example of single-stage revision of grossly infected tumor endoprosthesis. (B) No signs of infection 10 months later. (*From* Tsuchiya H, Shirai T, Nishida H, et al. Innovative antimicrobial coating of titanium implants with iodine. J Orthop Sci 2012;17(5):599; with permission.)

methyl methacrylate also allows for a wider variety of antibiotics to be used, because there is no exothermic reaction. The group found that antibiotic was released from the hydrogel within 96 hours, with a peak release between 2 and 4 hours. By coloring the hydrogel with methylene blue, the group was able to show the entire bone surface throughout the canal was contacted by the hydrogel, thus presumably treated with antibiotic. Last, comparison of hydrogel with and without antimicrobials showed "remarkable inhibition" of biofilm formation and of planktonic bacterial growth, compared with the hydrogel alone.[19]

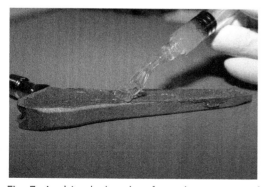

Fig. 7. Applying hydrogel to femoral component of total hip replacement. (*Adapted from* Romanò CL, Scarponi S, Gallazzi E, et al. Antibacterial coating of implants in orthopaedics and trauma: a classification proposal in an evolving panorama. J Orthop Surg Res 2015;10(1):157; with permission.)

SUMMARY

Prosthetic bacterial infections remain a challenging problem in orthopedic surgery. In this section, the authors reviewed passive surface modifications, such as alterations of nanoscale topography and the surface chemistry of metallic surfaces. They also reviewed active surface modifications, such as covalently attached host defense proteins and anodized iodine ions. Finally, the authors explored the use of surface treatments that release antibiotics such as methyl methacrylate and hydrogels. These approaches have varying advantages and disadvantages. Nevertheless, it is clear that modifications of implants may provide new opportunities to reduce the incidence of potentially devastating periprosthetic infections.

PART 2: BIOPRINTING IN ORTHOPEDIC SURGERY
Three-Dimensional Printing with Cells and Creating Tissues

As 3D printing and the use of well-established materials, such as polymers, metals, and simple composites for medical models, surgical guides, and permanent implantables, become increasingly commonplace (along with their chemically and physically modified surface variants) and improve patient care and reduce costs, new medical 3D printing technologies are beginning to emerge: tissue regenerative, acellular advanced biomaterial 3D printing, and live cell and tissue bioprinting. Objects fabricated using these advanced materials and processes go beyond imitating anatomic form and/or imparting structural support: they emulate the biological function of tissues they are replacing and may even transform into tissues indistinguishable, in both form and function, from the native biology.

Unlike traditional additive manufacturing nomenclature that defines distinct additive technologies based on the process used, such as fused deposition modeling, powder bed fusion (laser or electron beam), jetting, stereolithography, direct extrusion, "bioprinting" does not refer to a specific process or class of hardware. Rather, the term "bioprinting" generally refers to any additive manufacturing process that uses live cells or living tissue fragments during fabrication.[20] Thus, if the manufacturing process being used is jetting or direct extrusion, but the feedstock materials contain live cells, those processes can be generally referred to as "bioprinting." Unfortunately, the term "bioprinting" is still frequently used to incorrectly refer to medical 3D printing in general. The distinction is important because, although there are similarities among all medical 3D printing, the processing requirements, materials, manufacturing facilities, testing, utilization, sterilization, and regulatory aspects of bioprinted products, each of which are deserving of extended discussion, vary significantly from their nonliving counterparts.

Bioprinting Criteria

Bioprinting criteria can be divided into 3 major categories: 3D printing, structure, and cell encapsulation, illustrated in **Fig. 8**. The use of live cells in the manufacturing process places significant restrictions on the type of 3D printing platforms that can be used for bioprinting.

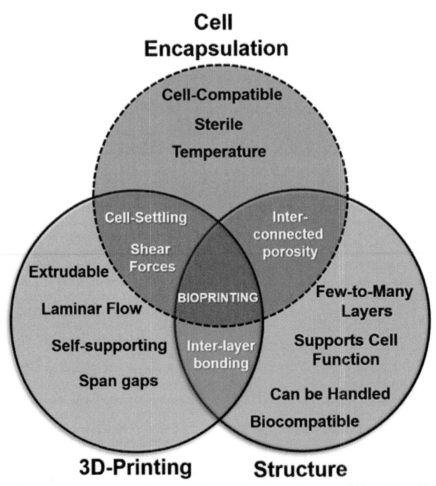

Fig. 8. The 3D printing, structure, and cell encapsulation criteria required for successful bioprinting. Note that the cell-encapsulation criteria are not required for advanced biomaterial (acelluar) 3D printing. (*Adapted from* Jakus AE, Rutz AL, Shah RN. Advancing the field of 3D biomaterial printing. Biomed Mater 2016;11(1):014102; with permission.)

Because of the sensitivity of cells to heat, radiation, and mechanical forces, bioprinting is almost exclusively restricted to material deposition-based rather than energy-based processes (powder-bed sintering or vat-based photo-cross-linking). Among the deposition-based approaches, including jetting[21] and nozzle-extrusion, which consists of the application of mechanical or pneumatic pressure to drive material out of a syringe or syringelike cartridge through a high-gauge nozzle, nozzle-extrusion is becoming increasingly dominant[20] due to its simplicity, scalability, versatility, speed, relative gentleness on live cells, and most significantly, increasing number of bio functional matrix materials compatible with the process.[22]

Of utmost importance is that the encapsulated cells and resulting bioprinted construct remain viable before, during, and after fabrication, requiring that the selective cell type be able to be cryogenically stored before use or be expanded into the required cell numbers for bioprinting soon after being isolated from their host. Those cells must remain viable as they are mixed into a cell-compatible matrix material (more in later discussion) and must survive the shear forces incurred during the 3D printing process. This must all be done at or near physiologic temperature, pH, and so forth, while also maintaining sterility. This latter point is especially important, because unlike traditional materials, such as metals and polymers, that can be sterilized using a variety of established, regulatory approved thermal, chemical, and radiative processes, bioprinted constructs cannot, as these processes would kill the comprising cells and destroy the construct.

In addition to maintaining the cytocompatibility of the cell-encapsulated materials before and during 3D printing, the cell-matrix material must also be able to be 3D printed in such a way that emulates the target tissue or organ structure. Therefore, the deposited material must be self-supporting upon deposition and be able to span gaps, producing interconnected porosity. Objects must also be transported to be surgically used. These usage criteria require that they be robust enough to be handled, transported, and surgically implemented without damaging the 3D-printed structure.

Cells Used for Bioprinting

Perhaps one of the most significant factors that differentiate bioprinting from traditional medical 3D printing is the type of materials used: live cells and the material matrices in which they are encapsulated, collectively referred to as bio-inks.[20,23] Unlike common 2D and simple 3D cell cultures, which require relatively few cells, bioprinting requires many millions if not billions of cells to be effective for most applications. As an example, an adult human is composed of more than 10 trillion individual cells,[24] and an adult liver alone contains more than 100 million cells per gram of tissue[25]; a typical liver weighs on average 1500 g, that is, 150 billion cells. That number comprises a variety of distinct and intermediate cell types and distinct structures, such as vasculature as well as bile duct networks.[26] Even if the goal is to bioprint a small fraction of a liver, the total number of cells required is exorbitant, as is the cellular density within the matrix material.

With such large numbers of functional cells required to effectively bioprint a piece of tissue, a major challenge becomes cell production and sourcing. The 5 major cell classes include: lines, primary, embryonic stem, adult stem, and induced pluripotent stem (iPS) (Fig. 9). Cell lines are easy to obtain, expand, and 3D print due to their physical robustness. However, cell lines are not representative of native cells in neither form nor function and are not clinically translatable. Primary cells, although the most representative of the 5 classes of cells, are difficult to store, source, and expand to sufficient numbers. Stem cells on the other hand are proliferative, relatively robust (suitable for 3D printing), and can be directed down certain tissue and subtissue lineages. Although embryonic stem cells have been successfully bioprinted,[27] they have generally fallen out of favor due to their limited availability. Adult stem cells, such as mesenchymal or adipose stem cells, MSCs and ASCs, respectively, are easily sourced, highly proliferative, and robust and can be directed toward a variety of cell types, making them suitable for select tissue targets, including adipose, muscle, and bone, among others. A recently demonstrated, new class of stem cells, iPS cells,[28] hold promise for being an effective source of cells for bioinks and bioprinting. As iPS technology improves, this class of cell and its derivative cell types are becoming easier and cheaper to obtain, but a foundation for their clinical use, unlike MSCs and ASCs, is still being established.

Matrix Materials Used for Bioprinting

The matrix materials used in the creation of bioinks are almost exclusively hydrogels, greater than 90% by weight water with minority polymeric network.[23] The types of materials used for the polymeric component of the hydrogel

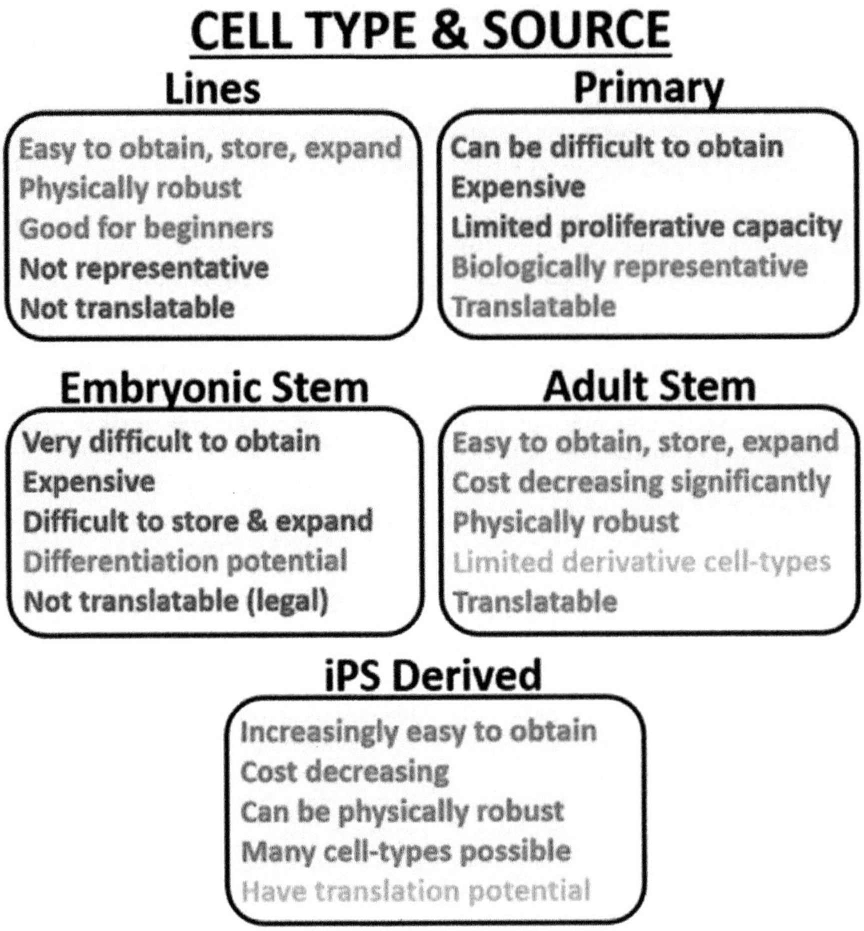

CELL TYPE & SOURCE

Lines

Easy to obtain, store, expand
Physically robust
Good for beginners
Not representative
Not translatable

Primary

Can be difficult to obtain
Expensive
Limited proliferative capacity
Biologically representative
Translatable

Embryonic Stem

Very difficult to obtain
Expensive
Difficult to store & expand
Differentiation potential
Not translatable (legal)

Adult Stem

Easy to obtain, store, expand
Cost decreasing significantly
Physically robust
Limited derivative cell-types
Translatable

iPS Derived

Increasingly easy to obtain
Cost decreasing
Can be physically robust
Many cell-types possible
Have translation potential

Fig. 9. Categories of cell types used for bioprinting and post–3D printing cell additions. Text colors denote prospect for clinical translation for particular characteristic: green = positive, red = limited, yellow = moderate.

are listed in Fig. 10 and can be separated into 2 major classes: naturally derived and synthetically derived. Naturally derived materials include those derived from plants, animals, fungus, and so forth and are primarily protein based (mammalian derived) or polysaccharide based (plant or fungus derived), whereas synthetically derived materials are based on synthetic chemistry, which can include synthetically produced peptides and peptide emulants, such as 3D-printable peptide amphiphiles.[29] Natural and synthetic materials may also be combined to create hybrid materials that may have advantages over each of their pure components.[22,23]

Much of bioprinting research to date has been performed using bioinks comprising cell lines and nonmammalian, natural materials, such as alginate, cellulose, and chitosan, due to their availability and low cost as well as their 3D printability. Despite being easy to work with, nonmammalian natural materials have limited cytocompatibility in vitro and typically elicit immune responses in vivo.[30] Mammalian-derived materials, on the other hand, such as collagen, gelatin (denatured collagen), and other pure extracellular matrix components, such as fibrin, laminin, hyaluronic acid, as well as tissue- and organ-specific decellularized extracellular matrices, are significantly more biofunctional and readily translatable than their nonmammalian counterparts.[23] Mammalian-derived materials, however, are generally more expensive and challenging to work with, although significant advances have been recently made related to the development of bioinks comprising mammalian-based materials, a necessary step for bioprinting technologies to be fully translated to the clinic.

Numerous approaches to bioprinting clinically relevant bioinks have been developed in recent years. One approach is to partially, physically cross-link thermoresponsive hydrogels, such as those based on gelatin, immediately before 3D printing, such that they are in an extrudable yet

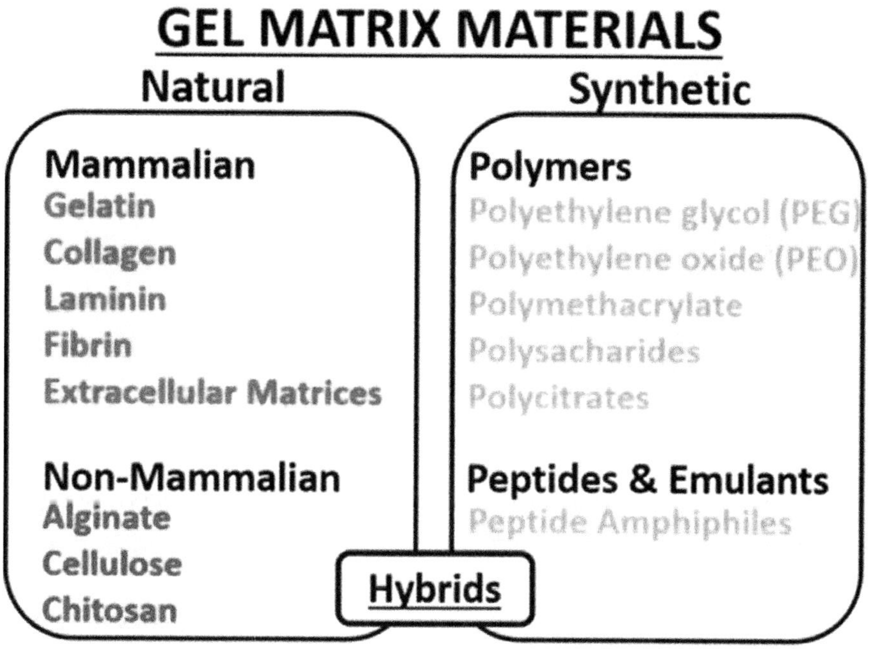

GEL MATRIX MATERIALS
Natural   Synthetic

Mammalian
Gelatin
Collagen
Laminin
Fibrin
Extracellular Matrices

Non-Mammalian
Alginate
Cellulose
Chitosan

Polymers
Polyethylene glycol (PEG)
Polyethylene oxide (PEO)
Polymethacrylate
Polysacharides
Polycitrates

Peptides & Emulants
Peptide Amphiphiles

Hybrids

Fig. 10. Categories and select examples of naturally and synthetically derived matrix materials for cell encapsulation and bioink synthesis. Text colors denote prospect for clinical translation: green = positive, red = limited, yellow = moderate.

self-supporting form, followed by full physical cross-linking at physiologic temperatures. This process was recently demonstrated by Laronda and Rutz and colleagues[31] and used to create functional, bioprosthetic mouse ovaries. Rutz and colleagues[22] also demonstrated a universal, 2-step chemical crosslinking approach based on polyethylene glycol that allows for successful encapsulation of numerous cell types in a variety of matrix materials while maintaining the ability to 3D-print complex structures, the *PEGX* method.

Various Approaches to Tissue Fabrication via Three-Dimensional Printing
Re-creating the smallest capillary networks, large vessels, stratified cell types, chemical gradients, cortices, and medullar regions all at once is a daunting task, but is it necessary to imitate a tissue or organ with such precision? Or is it enough to emulate the form, composition, and function just enough such that, once implanted or conditioned in vitro, the bioprinted object can mature and become a fully functioning unit? These respective, *imitative* and *emulative*, approaches are the 2 primary schools of thought when it comes to bioprinting tissues and organs (Fig. 11). Creating a fully functioning tissue unit or organ directly on a 3D printer would be ideal. However, because of the complexity of tissues and organs, it is simply not yet possible to directly fabricate a fully imitative tissue or organ. Most current bioprinting efforts take the emulative approach, relying on the intelligence and dynamic nature of biology to remodel and refine the original structure.

There is a third *transformative* approach that has only recently been made possible due to the development of new, advanced 3D-printable biomaterials (see **Fig. 11**). These materials, 3D-printed without cells or stimulatory growth factors, are highly bioactive due to their physical properties and induce tissue formation upon implantation. The recently developed *3D-Painting*[32] approach is one such technology that encompasses advanced biomaterials, such as *Hyperelastic Bone* (hard tissue regenerative),[33] *3D-Graphene* (electrically conductive and neuro regenerative),[34] *Tissue Papers* (organ-specific),[35] and others. 3D-Painting is a distinct process and is characterized by the room-temperature deposition and immediate solidification of highly particle-loaded suspension, *3D-Paints*. With no live cells or tissues used in the 3D printing process, 3D-Painting is technically not bioprinting, but this transformative approach can potentially be used to achieve results similar to bioprinted structures.

Overall Perspective on Cell and Tissue Bioprinting
Bioprinting technology has advanced at an incredible rate in the past 5 years primarily

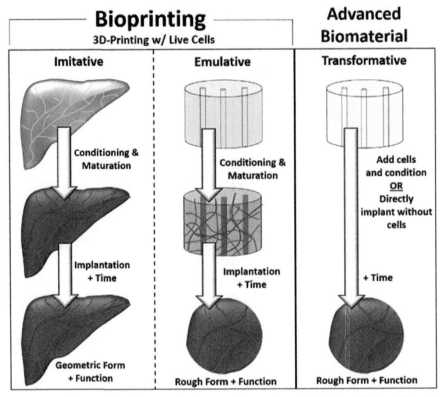

Fig. 11. A representative example of 3 categorical approaches to tissue fabrication with liver. Bioprinting can be divided into 2 subcategories: imitative and emulative. Acellular advanced biomaterials can be used in a transformative approach to achieve similar results as those achieved in the emulative process.

because of the increasing availability and reduced price of clinically relevant cell types and biomaterials, the wider availability and selection of bioprinting compatible hardware, and increased awareness and education around the subject. At the time of this writing, there are currently no FDA-cleared bioprinted products on the market, but this will likely change in the coming several years as quality control and manufacturing of bioprinted tissues are improved upon and become more reliable. As traditional medical 3D printing technologies become standard for many clinical applications, bioprinting and regenerative biomaterial technologies will eventually transform large sectors of the health care industry, not only by introducing new treatments but also by influencing the forms in treatment to be delivered, paid for, and evaluated.

REFERENCES

1. Ha KY, Chung YG, Ryoo SJ. Adherence and biofilm formation of Staphylococcus epidermidis and Mycobacterium tuberculosis on various spinal implants. Spine 2005;30:38–43.

2. Romanò CL, Scarponi S, Gallazzi E, et al. Antibacterial coating of implants in orthopaedics and trauma: a classification proposal in an evolving panorama. J Orthop Surg Res 2015; 10:157.

3. Gallo J, Holinka M, Moucha CS. Antibacterial surface treatment for orthopaedic implants. Int J Mol Sci 2014;15:13849–80.

4. Gristina AG, Naylor P, Myrvik Q, et al. Infections from biomaterials and implants: a race for the surface. Medical Progress Through Technology 1988; 14(3-4):205–24.

5. Yount NY, Yeaman MR. Emerging themes and therapeutic prospects for anti-infective peptides. Annu Rev Pharmacol Toxicol 2012;52:337–60.

6. Pogodin S, Hasan J, Baulin VA, et al. Biophysical model of bacterial cell interactions with nanopatterned cicada wing surfaces. Biophys J 2013;104: 835–40.

7. Anselme K, Davidson P, Popa AM, et al. The interaction of cells and bacteria with surfaces structured at the nanometre scale. Acta Biomater 2010;6: 3824–46.

8. Chen S, Li Y, Cheng YF. Nanopatterning of steel by one-step anodization for anti-adhesion of bacteria. Sci Rep 2017;7:5326.

9. Singh AV, Vyas V, Patil R, et al. Quantitative characterization of the influence of the nanoscale morphology of nanostructured surfaces on bacterial adhesion and biofilm formation. PLoS One 2011;6:e25029.

10. Dickson MN, Liang EI, Rodriguez LA, et al. Nanopatterned polymer surfaces with bactericidal properties. Biointerphases 2015;10:021010.

11. Campoccia D, Montanaro L, Arciola CR. A review of the clinical implications of anti-infective biomaterials and infection-resistant surfaces. Biomaterials 2013;34:8018–29.

12. De Brucker K, Delattin N, Robijns S, et al. Derivatives of the mouse cathelicidin-related antimicrobial peptide (CRAMP) inhibit fungal and bacterial biofilm formation. Antimicrob Agents Chemother 2014;58:5395–404.

13. Shirai T, Shimizu T, Ohtani K, et al. Antibacterial iodine-supported titanium implants. Acta Biomater 2011;7:1928–33.

14. Tsuchiya H, Shirai T, Nishida H, et al. Innovative antimicrobial coating of titanium implants with iodine. J Orthop Sci 2012;17:595–604.

15. Inoue D, Kabata T, Ohtani K, et al. Inhibition of biofilm formation on iodine-supported titanium implants. Int Orthop 2017;41:1093–9.

16. Engesaeter LB, Lie SA, Espehaug B, et al. Antibiotic prophylaxis in total hip arthroplasty: effects of antibiotic prophylaxis systemically and in bone cement on the revision rate of 22,170 primary hip replacements followed 0-14 years in the Norwegian Arthroplasty Register. Acta Orthop Scand 2003;74.644 51.

17. Gogia JS, Meehan JP, Di Cesare PE, et al. Local antibiotic therapy in osteomyelitis. Semin Plast Surg 2009;23:100–7.

18. Neut D, Hendriks JGE, van Horn JR, et al. Pseudomonas aeruginosa biofilm formation and slime excretion on antibiotic-loaded bone cement. Acta Orthop 2005;76:109–14.

19. Drago L, Boot W, Dimas K, et al. Does implant coating with antibacterial-loaded hydrogel reduce bacterial colonization and biofilm formation in vitro? Clin Orthop Relat Res 2014;472:3311–23.

20. Jakus AE, Rutz AL, Shah RN. Advancing the field of 3D biomaterial printing. Biomed Mater 2016;11(1): 014102.

21. Gao G, Schilling AF, Hubbell K, et al. Improved properties of bone and cartilage tissue from 3D inkjet-bioprinted human mesenchymal stem cells by simultaneous deposition and photocrosslinking in PEG-GelMA. Biotechnol Lett 2015;37(11):2349–55.

22. Rutz AL, Hyland KE, Jakus AE, et al. A multimaterial bioink method for 3D printing tunable, cell-compatible hydrogels. Adv Mater 2015;27(9): 1607–14.

23. Rutz AL, Lewis PL, Shah RN. Toward next-generation bioinks: tuning material properties pre- and post-printing to optimize cell viability. MRS Bull 2017;42(8):563–70.

24. Bianconi E, Piovesan A, Facchin F, et al. An estimation of the number of cells in the human body. Ann Hum Biol 2013;40(6):463–71.

25. Wilson ZE, Rostami-Hodjegan A, Burn JL, et al. Inter-individual variability in levels of human microsomal protein and hepatocellularity per gram of liver. Br J Clin Pharmacol 2003;56(4): 433–40.

26. Lewis PL, Shah RN. 3D printing for liver tissue engineering: current approaches and future challenges. Curr Transplant Rep 2016;3(1):100–8.

27. Xu F, Sridharan B, Wang S, et al. Embryonic stem cell bioprinting for uniform and controlled size embryoid body formation. Biomicrofluidics 2011; 5(2):022207.

28. Shi Y, Inoue H, Wu JC, et al. Induced pluripotent stem cell technology: a decade of progress. Nat Rev Drug Discov 2016;16:115.

29. Yan M, Lewis PL, Shah RN. Tailoring nanostructure and bioactivity of 3D-printable hydrogels with self-assemble peptides amphiphile (PA) for promoting bile duct formation. Biofabrication 2018;10(3): 035010.

30. Rezaa Mohammadi M, Rodrigez S, Cao R, et al. Immune response to subcutaneous implants of alginate microcapsules. Mater Today 2018;5(7, Part 3). 15580–5.

31. Laronda MM, Rutz AL, Xiao S, et al. A bioprosthetic ovary created using 3D printed microporous scaffolds restores ovarian function in sterilized mice. Nat Commun 2017;8:15261.

32. Jakus AE, Geisendorfer NR, Lewis PL, et al. 3D-printing porosity: a new approach to creating elevated porosity materials and structures. Acta Biomater 2018;72:94–109.

33. Jakus AE, Rutz AL, Jordan SW, et al. Hyperelastic "bone": a highly versatile, growth factor-free, osteoregenerative, scalable, and surgically friendly biomaterial. Sci Transl Med 2016;8(358):358ra127.

34. Jakus AE, Secor EB, Rutz AL, et al. Three-dimensional printing of high-content graphene scaffolds for electronic and biomedical applications. ACS Nano 2015;9(4):4636–48.

35. Jakus AE, Laronda MM, Rashedi AS, et al. "Tissue papers" from organ-specific decellularized extracellular matrices. Adv Funct Mater 2017;27(34): 1700992.

A Randomized Study of Exercise and Fitness Trackers in Obese Patients After Total Knee Arthroplasty

Webb A. Smith, PhD[a],*,
Audrey Zucker-Levin, PhD, PT, MBA[b],
William M. Mihalko, MD, PhD[c], Michael Williams, PT[d],
Mark Loftin, PhD[e], James G. Gurney, PhD[f]

KEYWORDS

- Total knee arthroplasty • Exercise intervention • Fitness • Quality of life • Fitness trackers

KEY POINTS

- Functional limitations and impaired quality of life often persist in obese patients after total knee arthroplasty (TKA).
- A 16-week individualized home-based aerobic and resistance training program improved function and quality of life in obese patients with TKA.
- Fitness trackers do not appear to have additional benefit when compared with a tailored exercise program alone.

INTRODUCTION

Osteoarthritis (OA) is a serious joint disease affecting more than 27 million adults in the United States.[1] Incidence and prevalence of OA have steadily increased over the past 20 years accentuating this serious public health concern.[2] Both the severity of the disease and the number living with OA make it one of the leading causes of long-term disability.[3,4] Clinical care of OA has met the increased demands through improved care and management, which in those with severe debilitating disease now routinely includes total knee arthroplasty (TKA).

Most patients report the ability to return to regular activities, such as walking, hiking, and swimming, with some patients even returning to sports like golf, tennis, and jogging after TKA.[5,6] However, it appears that obesity and physical inactivity and increased joint loads, which are major contributors to the development and progression of OA, remain

Disclosure Statement: The authors have no financial disclosures or relationships with companies or manufacturers that would benefit from the results of this study.
This work was supported by the FedEx Institute of Technology at the University of Memphis.
[a] Department of Pediatrics, University of Tennessee Health Science Center, 50 North Dunlap Street, Room 453R, Memphis, TN 38103, USA; [b] Department of Physical Therapy, College of Health Professions, University of Tennessee Health Science Center, 930 Madison Avenue, Suite 636, Memphis, TN 38163, USA; [c] Joint Graduate Program in Biomedical Engineering, Department of Orthopedic Surgery and Biomedical Engineering, Campbell Clinic, University of Tennessee Health Science Center, 956 Court Avenue, Memphis, TN 38163, USA; [d] Department of Physical Therapy, Campbell Clinic Orthopaedics, 1400 South Germantown Road, Germantown, TN 38138, USA; [e] Department of Exercise Science, School of Applied Sciences, George Street University House, University, MS 38677, USA; [f] Division of Epidemiology, Biostatistics and Environmental Health, School of Public Health, University of Memphis, 228 Robison Hall, Memphis, TN 38152, USA
* Corresponding author.
E-mail address: wsmith74@uthsc.edu

problematic after TKA. Despite the ability to return to these activities, it appears that poor exercise habits that preceded surgery return following the initial recovery period.[7] Most studies indicate that TKA does not result in decreased body weight, in fact body weight often increases after the surgical procedure.[8–11]

The persistence of low activity levels may result in long-term functional abilities that are significantly compromised. Thus, functional recovery, such as general mobility, gait mechanics, walking endurance, ability to walk stairs, freedom from pain, and quality of life, may not be as thorough and lasting as could be expected. It has commonly been assumed by medical professionals and reported by patients that obesity and physical inactivity were a result of OA and the common symptoms of pain and physical limitation. More recently, it has been suggested that obesity and physical inactivity should be treated as separate medical issues because they do not appear to improve with the restored function and reduced pain following TKA.[9,10,12]

The role of exercise therapy has received relatively little attention outside of short-duration interventions and injury-specific postoperative rehabilitation. Exercise interventions, including both aerobic and strength training, have been shown to improve aerobic fitness, mobility, coordination, and body composition; increase muscle mass and bone density; and reduce depression and anxiety in many clinical populations,[13] all of which are relevant for obese patients after a TKA. However, based on the extant literature, few post-rehabilitation exercise interventions have been formally conducted and evaluated in patients with TKA.

Preoperative and early postoperative studies, including exercise intervention, focusing on rehabilitation of the injured area, have shown that leg strength and improving leg strength was predictive of better function 1 year after surgery.[14–16] In one of the only exercise interventions in patients more than 1 year from TKA, LaStayo and colleagues[6] conducted a pilot study using a 12-week supervised strength training program designed to improve muscle strength in the quadriceps and reported significant increases in strength and mobility. These preliminary data offer promise that exercise interventions can improve the long-term function and outcomes from TKA.

Any potential exercise intervention in obese patients with TKA must balance improving physical fitness levels and minimizing wear on the prosthesis. Although there have been few studies evaluating the biomechanical stress that common activities place on the knee joint in obese patients, post joint replacement exercise recommendations are available based on a survey of 54 members of Hip and Knee Society who provided their expert opinion on common sporting activities. Activities that were recommended consisted of exercises such as stationary cycling, swimming, walking, golf, low-impact aerobics, weight machines, and dancing.[17] In addition to minimizing wear on the joint, consideration has to be given to motivation to become physically active. Patients with OA and obese patients with TKA are routinely advised to become more physically active and lose weight before surgery. However, reports indicate that only approximately one-third of patients are successful at increasing physical activity and ultimately reducing body weight.[18] Howarth and colleagues[19] assessed barriers to weight loss in obese patients with knee OA, and although 29% reported pain as major barrier, nearly 90% reported lack of motivation to be the largest barrier to weight loss. For an exercise intervention to be successful, these barriers must be carefully considered in the exercise program.

Activity trackers are widely used by millions of consumers to track and increase physical activity. Although there are many anecdotal reports that fitness-tracking devices increase physical activity and motivation, there is little published evidence. The evidence available is encouraging and suggests the devices alone may be enough to positively influence activity patterns.[20,21] The incorporation of fitness-tracking technology in conjunction with tailored interventions offer an intriguing way to provide low-cost and sustainable interventions to increase physical function and activity levels.

This group of obese patients with TKA have additional barriers and deficits to a thorough recovery previously published.[22] We hypothesize these barriers and physical limitations could benefit from a tailored general fitness program at the 1-year follow-up visit when postsurgical rehabilitation is long completed and full healing should have occurred. The primary outcomes of this project were to assess the impact of a 16-week home-based exercise intervention in obese patients with knee replacement with comparison of additional benefits from the fitness tracker.

METHODS

Experimental Approach to the Problem

After signing the informed consent, participants were randomly assigned using a dual random number matrix procedure to 1 of 2 intervention groups. Both intervention groups received a 16-week tailored home-based exercise program based on the American College of Sports Medicine (ACSM) guidelines for exercise prescription.[23] In addition to the tailored exercise program, participants in one of the intervention arms received a fitness tracker. The fitness tracker, in theory, provided additional motivation through feedback on amount of exercise completed and progress toward goals. Participants in both intervention arms were assessed at baseline, after the 8-week intervention (week 9) and after the 16-week intervention (week 17).

Subjects

Sixty obese patients who were 10 to 18 months post TKA volunteered to complete surveys and participate in a functional assessment. Patients were required to have medical clearance to participate in exercise testing and intervention. Patients were identified and recruited from surgical follow-up clinics at a large health science center and privately based orthopedic practice. Before consent, each participant was prescreened for eligibility by a research nurse coordinator by phone (**Fig. 1**). Participants were informed of all procedures, potential risks, and benefits associated with the study with procedures approved by the Institutional Review Boards for Human Subjects research at the University of Tennessee Health Sciences Center and the University of Memphis and written informed consent was obtained from each. Final eligibility was verified through health and medical history and a physical activity survey at the initial clinic visit.

Baseline testing was completed on 60 patients (39 women; 21 men) who were randomly assigned to an exercise-only group or exercise and fitness tracker group. There were no statistically significant differences between groups at baseline (**Table 1**).

Measurements

Anthropometrics. Height and weight were collected without shoes using a calibrated digital clinic scale and a wall-mounted stadiometer. Body composition was measured using standardized skinfold measures developed by Jackson and Pollock and described in detail by the ACSM.[23] Skinfolds were measured with Lange skinfold caliper (Beta Technology, Santa Cruz, CA) recorded at the chest, abdomen, and thigh in men and triceps, suprailiac crest, and thigh in women. Sum of skinfolds measured was used to calculated percentage body fat using 2-stage

predictive equations by first calculating body density and then body fat percentage.[23] Body mass index (BMI) was calculated by dividing kilograms of body weight by height in meters squared. Waist and hip circumference was measured using a Gulick II tape measure at the narrowest point between the umbilicus and the xiphoid process and the widest point between umbilicus and the knee, respectively.

Physical function. Heart rate, blood pressure, and respirations were measured following a 5-minute quiet seated rest period. Walk endurance was measured using the 6-minute walk test (6 MW), which consists of continuous walking at a self-selected pace in accordance with the American Thoracic Society guidelines.[24] During the 6 MW, participants were encouraged to walk as quickly as possible for 6 minutes on the designated walk path. Participants could stop and rest as needed during the test; however, the test timer did not stop. The distance walked (meters) in 6 minutes was recorded for each participant. Expected normative walk distances were based on previously published predictive equations in age-matched and gender-matched healthy adults.[25]

Passive and active range of motion at the knee was measured by a licensed physical therapist using a goniometer. Participants were instructed to flex and extend the knee actively as far as possible, and passive measures were recorded by the physical therapist at the terminal range in degrees. Knee extension strength was measured using a handheld dynamometer (Chatillon DFE; Lloyd Instruments, Largo, FL). The participants were seated with the knee positioned at 60° and the dynamometer was placed 20 cm below the tibial tuberosity. The participant was instructed to extend the lower leg against the dynamometer as hard as possible. Three trials were performed on each leg with 1-minute rest between trials. Predicted strength values were based on previously published gender-based normative ranges in healthy adults.[26]

Self-reported knee function and health-related quality of life. The Western Ontario and McMaster University Osteoarthritis Index (WOMAC) was used to assess pain, function, and quality of life in patients with OA of the knee.[27] Responses to each question range from 0, indicating none, to 4, indicating severe; thus, higher scores on the composite or subscales indicate worse pain, stiffness, or function. WOMAC scoring yields 1 composite (0–96) and

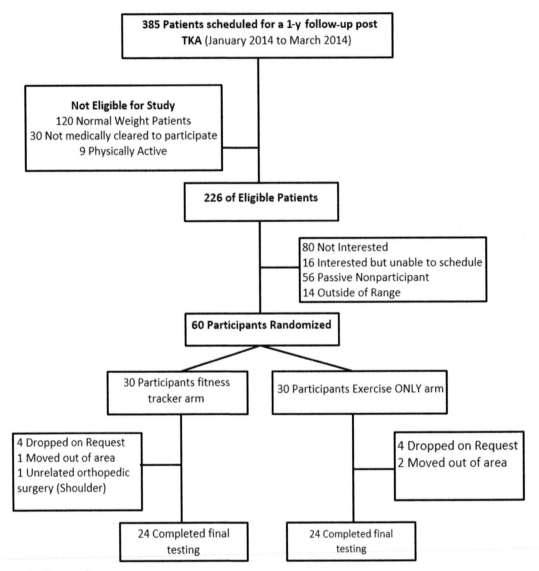

Fig. 1. Consort diagram.

3 subscales: pain (0–20), stiffness (0–8), and physical function (0–68). The composite and subscales have been shown to have reasonable validity (Spearman correlations from 0.63 to 0.67) and reliability (Cronbach alphas from 0.86 to 0.95).[28,29]

Health-related quality of life was assessed using the Medical Outcomes Study Short-Form 36 version 2 (SF36v2).[30,31] The SF36v2 is a widely used questionnaire designed to assess health-related quality of life. The survey is a generic health survey, which has been used in many populations, including obese and OA populations.[32] Scores were calculated for 8 health domains (mental health, role physical, physical function, vitality, social function, bodily pain, role emotional, and general health), the physical component summary (PCS) and mental component summary (MCS). Survey responses were summed to generate raw scores in each subscale and health domain and used to create general population norm-based scoring (t scores with a population mean of 50 and a standard deviation of 10) using previously prescribed methodology.[30,31] Scores were considered poor if the normalized scores (T-Scores) were less than 37, which corresponds to the lowest 10th percentile of the general population. Scores were considered to be average or better if the normalized scores (T-Scores) were greater than 48, which correspond to the greater than 40th percentile of the general population.

Table 1
Baseline group characteristics

Variable	Total (N = 48) n (%)	Fitness Tracker and Exercise (n = 24) n (%)	Exercise Only (n = 24) n (%)	
Men	21 (43.8)	10 (20.8)	11 (22.9)	
Smoker	3 (6.3)	2 (4.1)	1 (2.1)	
	Mean ± SD	Mean ± SD	Mean ± SD	P
Age, y	64.2 ± 8.9	63.9 ± 9.7	64.5 ± 8.2	.81
Height, cm	165.8 ± 11.1	166.9 ± 10.6	164.7 ± 11.7	.48
Weight, kg	101.8 ± 18.2	101.9 ± 16.8	101.7 ± 19.9	.97
BMI, kg/m^2	37.0 ± 5.4	36.4 ± 3.9	37.5 ± 6.5	.47
Skinfolds, mm	135.6 ± 20.6	131.9 ± 21.3	139.2 ± 19.5	.21
Waist to hip	0.90 ± 0.10	0.91 ± 0.09	0.89 ± 0.11	.24
HR, beats per minute	71.9 ± 5.9	71.6 ± 5.3	72.1 ± 6.5	.79
SBP, mm Hg	130.4 ± 8.9	129.3 ± 8.1	131.5 ± 9.6	.37
DBP, mm Hg	81.0 ± 4.5	80.3 ± 3.7	81.7 ± 5.2	.28

Abbreviations: BMI, body mass index; DBP, diastolic blood pressure; HR, heart rate; SBP, systolic blood pressure.

All testing was completed by the same clinical exercise physiologist, with the exception of lower extremity range of motion and the WOMAC index, which were completed by the same licensed physical therapist.

Intervention. All participants in the study received a 16-week home-based exercise program based on guidelines for exercise prescription from the ACSM.[23] The program included tailored resistance and aerobic training designed to be completed at home with no supervision and minimal equipment. The program was tailored to each individual and included weekly phone calls from the study exercise physiologist. The weekly phone calls were used to monitor compliance, assess the patient's progress, and modify the exercise prescription as needed.

The resistance training program consisted of 8 to 10 exercises. Each exercise was done for 1 set of 12 to 15 repetitions on 2 nonsuccessive days per week. The program was progressed over the phone by increasing the difficulty of the selected exercises and by increasing the volume of resistance training prescribed (number of sets and/or number of days per week) in a systematic and incremental manner. The loading on the affected knee joint was minimized with exercise selections in accordance with recommendations from the Knee Society Survey.[17]

The aerobic training program consisted of the patient's choice and availability of equipment of walking, cycling, or other low-impact options recommended by the Knee Society Survey.[17] Aerobic training began with 3 days per week for 20 minutes (or two 10-minute sessions) at a low-intensity walk (or alternative activity with equivalent intensity). The aerobic program was increased over the phone by progressively increasing duration to a maximum of 60 minutes, increasing intensity to a maximum of power walking (or alternative activity with equivalent intensity), and increasing number of sessions per week to a maximum of 5 days per week as tolerated. As with the resistance exercises, the aerobic training program was tailored for each individual based on the baseline functional assessment and progression was adjusted as needed based on patient feedback from weekly phone calls.

All participants received a demonstration of each exercise and an introduction to the forms and logs in the program at the end of the baseline functional assessment. During this education session, handouts were provided that included a visual depiction and written explanation of the prescribed exercise. In addition to the educational handouts, workout logs were provided so that the patient could record and track his or her workouts and provide comments. The workout logs were used as a reference during the weekly phone calls and to record compliance to the exercise program.

Each participant assigned to the fitness tracker study arm received additional motivational input via a commercially available Fitbit wireless fitness tracker (Fitbit Inc, San Francisco, CA) for use during the study (provided free of charge to the participant). The Fitbit wireless fitness tracker is a small device (about the size of an AA battery) that can be worn as a bracelet (Fitbit Flex), or clipped to a necklace, waistline or other clothing (Fitbit One). The device tracks and provides feedback on the number of steps taken, number of stairs climbed and estimates caloric expenditure.

Data analysis. The first analytical step was an evaluation of dropouts, comparisons of baseline characteristics, and evaluation of the impact of the fitness tracker on adherence to the exercise program. This was done with a 1-way analysis of variance comparing the adherence rates between the exercise-only group and exercise plus fitness tracker group. General linear models repeated measures procedures were used to compare the functional outcomes and quality-of-life measurements across the 3 intervention time points (pre, mid, and post) by treatment group. The Mauchly test was used to assess sphericity; where the assumption of sphericity was violated, a Huynh-Feldt correction was used. Significant main effects were evaluated with Bonferroni post hoc analysis to identify individual differences. Statistical significance was set with $\alpha = 0.05$. All data reduction, processing, and analysis for this project were generated using IBM SPSS Statistics software, version 22, 64-bit edition of the SPSS system for Windows (IBM Corporation, Armonk, NY).

RESULTS

Participants

Of the 60 patients randomized, 12 patients (20%) failed to complete the follow-up assessment, leaving 24 participants in the exercise and fitness-tracking group and 24 participants in the exercise-only group (see Fig. 1, Table 1). Of the 12 patients who did not return for follow-up testing, 7 were women, and none were smokers. Of the 6 participants who dropped out of the fitness tracker group, 1 patient had unrelated orthopedic surgery (shoulder), 1 patient lost his or her home and relocated, 2 patients withdrew (did not have time), and 2 patients started new jobs (travel). Of the 6 participants who dropped out of the exercise-only group, 2 patients withdrew (did not have time), 1 patient relocated out of state, 1 patient started a new job (travel), and 2 patients withdrew due to lack of interest. There were no statistically significant baseline differences in age ($P = .28$), BMI ($P = .14$), skinfold

thickness ($P = .58$), distance walked ($P = .98$), degrees of knee extension ($P = .55$), or self-reported pain ($P = .62$), function ($P = .89$), or stiffness ($P = .43$) between those who completed the study and those who did not complete the study.

Fitness Tracker

The fitness tracker failed to increase overall compliance with the exercise program. Among those who completed the study, average compliance with the prescribed exercise sessions was not different between fitness tracker and exercise group and exercise-only group (78.6 ± 8.5 vs 74.8 ± 11.0; $F [1, 50] = 1.80$, $P = .19$). During the informal interview regarding the device, 2 clear groups emerged. One group (16 patients) reported a positive impact of the device. This group enjoyed the feedback about their activity levels and were interested in the technology. This group took advantage of the Web site, e-mail reports, and the smart phone applications. The second group (12 patients) negatively viewed the device. The most common reason for not liking the device was they did not think the information was useful. In general, those in the group with negative feedback on the fitness tracker were not regular consumers of technology (ie, e-mail, Web sites, or text message) and did not use the smart phone applications or the Web sites. This group reported forgetting to wear the device frequently and not liking technology in general.

The fitness tracker had no statistically significant effect on any parameters tested, including vitals, anthropometrics, knee range of motion, strength, walk performance, or self-reported function or quality of life. Therefore, the remaining results are pooled estimates across the 2 intervention arms and present the average time main effects of the exercise program.

Vitals and Anthropometrics

Resting heart rate did not change significantly following 16 weeks of home-based exercise (Table 2). The exercise program did result in a statistically significant decrease in systolic ($\chi^2 [2] = 8.234$ $P = .016$, $F [1.812, 83.353] = 7.089$, $P = .01$) and diastolic blood pressure ($\chi^2 [2] = 11.301$ $P = .004$, $F [1.812, 79.378] = 11.721$, $P<.001$). For both systolic and diastolic blood pressure, analysis revealed significantly lower blood pressure from baseline to 8 weeks and 16 weeks but no differences between measurements at 8 and 16 weeks.

Patients did not significantly reduce body weight or BMI on average during the 16-week home-based exercise program. There were

Table 2
Effect of 16-week home-based exercise program on physical performance

	Baseline Mean ± SD	8 wk Mean ± SD	16 wk Mean ± SD	P
Resting vitals				
HR, bpm	71.8 ± 5.9	71.0 ± 5.9	71.3 ± 5.9	.48
SBP, mm Hg	130.0 ± 8.3	127.8 ± 7.8	126.7 ± 8.5	.002[a]
DBP, mm Hg	80.7 ± 4.3	78.5 ± 4.1	78.2 ± 4.0	<.001[a]
Anthropometrics				
Body weight, kg	100.9 ± 18.1	100.2 ± 18.0	100.4 ± 18.2	.13
BMI, kg/m^2	36.4 ± 4.7	36.1 ± 4.8	36.2 ± 5.0	.18
Sum of skinfolds, mm	135.6 ± 21.0	120.9 ± 21.0	113.3 ± 21.0	<.001[a]
Waist to hip	0.90 ± 0.10	0.89 ± 0.10	0.88 ± 0.09	.001[a]
Active knee range of motion, degrees				
Extension, lacking full extension		—	—	—
TKA, degrees	2.2 ± 4.0	1.3 ± 3.7	1.0 ± 3.8	.003[a]
Non-TKA, degrees	1.9 ± 5.4	1.1 ± 4.8	0.9 ± 5.8	.041[a]
Flexion	—	—	—	—
TKA, degrees	119.0 ± 9.7	119.3 ± 9.1	120.3 ± 9.1	.20
Non-TKA, degrees	121.3 ± 10.8	123.0 ± 11.4	123.6 ± 10.8	.02[a]
Knee extensor strength				
TKA, kg	57.5 ± 19.4	69.2 ± 18.4	73.8 ± 20.9	<.001[a]
Non-TKA, kg	56.9 ± 17.2	68.7 ± 17.6	73.6 ± 21.4	<.001[a]
Six-minute walk				
Distance, m	310.5 ± 77.0	369.4 ± 80.9	378.3 ± 84.5	<.001[a]

Abbreviations: BMI, body mass index; DBP, diastolic blood pressure; HR, heart rate; SBP, systolic blood pressure; TKA, total knee arthroplasty.
[a] $P<.05$.

statically significant reductions in sum of skinfolds (χ^2 [2] = 20.764, $P<.001$, F [1.529, 70.325] = 152.606, $P<.001$) and waist-to-hip ratio (χ^2 [2] = 9.571 P = .008, F [1.773, 81.540] = 8.114, P = .001). Sum of skinfold measurements declined throughout the study period, with significant differences between each time point. Waist-to-hip ratio was significantly lower from baseline to 16 weeks and from 8 weeks to 16 weeks (see Table 2).

Knee Range of Motion and Extensor Strength
Active knee extension values were slightly short of full extension on the TKA and non-TKA leg. Statistically significant improvements were observed in the TKA (χ^2 [2] = 5.515 P = .063, F [2, 92] = 6.313, P = .003) and non-TKA knee (χ^2 [2] = 7.975 P = .019, F [1.823, 83.861] = 3.423, P = .041). These improvements in range of motion in TKA and non-TKA legs are noted only from baseline to 16-week measurements. Active knee flexion values did not significantly improve

in the TKA knee (χ^2 [2] = 12.936 P = .002, F [1.685, 77.506] = 1.673, P = .198) but did significantly improve in the non-TKA knee (χ^2 [2] = 9.199 P = .010, F [1.783, 82.031] = 4.278, P = .021). Similar to the results from knee extension, differences in knee flexion in the non-TKA leg were noted only from baseline to 16-week follow-up.

Knee extensor strength showed notable improvements following 16 weeks of home-based exercise. Knee extension strength in the both TKA (χ^2 [2] = 18.053 $P<.001$, F [1.577, 72.525] = 55.741, $P<.001$) and non-TKA (χ^2 [2] = 3.689 P = .158, F [2, 92] = 49.586, $P<.001$) legs improved significantly. TKA and not-TKA strength measurements improved throughout the study with significant differences noted between each time point (see Table 2).

Six-Minute Test Walk Performance
Total distance walked during 6 minutes improved on average by 67.5 m (percent change

of 21.7%) from baseline to the final assessment, which represents a clinically significant improvement in walk distance. These improvements in walk distance were also statistically significant (χ^2 [2] = 8.096 P = .017, F [1.813, 81.578] = 47.886, $P<.001$). Significant improvements in walk distance were observed from baseline to 8 weeks and 16 weeks but not between 8-week and 16-week measurements.

Self-Reported Knee Function
WOMAC composite scores improved significantly (χ^2 [2] = 1.884 P = .390, F [2, 92] = 4.204, P = .018) (Table 3). The improvements in self-reported knee function were noted only from baseline to 8-week follow-up. These improvements in the WOMAC composite score appear to driven by improved perceptions of knee function. The knee function subscale of the WOMAC scale improved significantly (χ^2 [2] = 4.148 P = .126, F [2, 92] = 5.616, P = .005), whereas pain (χ^2 [2] = 1.124 P = .570, F [2, 92] = 2.40 P = −.097) and stiffness (χ^2 [2] = 0.142 P = .932, F [2, 92] = 1.461, P = .237) subscales did not improve significantly. The scores on the function subscale improved significantly from baseline to 8 weeks (P = .014).

Self-Reported Health-Related Quality of Life
PCS scores improved significantly across time (χ^2 [2] = 5.201 P = .074, F [2, 92] = 3.313 P = −.041). In addition, nonsignificant increases

in role physical (χ^2 [2] = 4.611 P = .100, F [2, 92] = 2.824 P = .065) and physical function (χ^2 [2] = 4.030, P = .133, F [2, 92] = 2.886 P = .061) subscales were observed. There were no substantive changes in scores on the MCS scores (χ^2 [2] = 12.493 P = .002, F [1.696, 77.998] = 1.625 P = .206), bodily pain (χ^2 [2] = 0.865 P = .649, F [2, 92] = 0.858 P = .427), or general health (χ^2 [2] = 7.520 P = .023, F [1.834, 84.375] = 0.679 P = .498) subscales.

DISCUSSION

The management of knee OA and its debilitating symptoms has advanced significantly in recent decades.[1,5] These advancements necessitate the evaluation of the outcomes after TKA. This is particularly important, specifically in the growing number of obese patients. Previous work has shown that obese patients are at greater risk of TKA and have worse outcomes after TKA. The results of this project show that a home-based exercise program in obese patients with TKA can improve knee extensor strength and walking distance. The results of this study also indicate that a 16-week home-based exercise program may improve patient perceptions of knee function and health-related quality of life. However, fitness tracking on average was not a significant motivational factor to enhance the effectiveness of the prescribed exercise program.

Table 3 Changes in health-related quality of life				
	Baseline Mean ± SD	8 wk Mean ± SD	16 wk Mean ± SD	P
Western Ontario and McMaster University Osteoarthritis Index				
Composite score	19.6 ± 14.4	16.6 ± 13.4	16.6 ± 14.0	.018[a]
Pain	3.3 ± 3.3	2.7 ± 2.8	2.9 ± 3.2	.097
Function	14.4 ± 12.1	11.3 ± 10.0	11.6 ± 10.2	.005[a]
Stiffness	2.5 ± 1.5	2.5 ± 1.5	2.2 ± 1.3	.237
SF-36 component scales[b]				
Physical component scale	40.7 ± 9.7	42.0 ± 8.9	43.3 ± 10.2	.041[a]
Mental component scale	56.1 ± 7.9	57.3 ± 7.5	55.2 ± 9.9	.206
SF-36 subscales[b]				
Physical function	54.2 ± 25.1	58.2 ± 23.7	59.4 ± 24.6	.061
Role physical	65.5 ± 27.9	69.4 ± 25.6	73.0 ± 28.4	.065
Bodily pain	62.9 ± 21.5	64.8 ± 20.8	66.2 ± 23.0	.427
General health	71.2 ± 16.3	73.6 ± 15.0	72.4 ± 15.7	.498

[a] $P<.05$.
[b] Normative scores (T-Scores).

This study demonstrates that a 16-week home-based exercise program is feasible and effective in improving strength and walk performance. Several studies have documented knee extensor strength weakness in patients with TKA, and most reports suggest a deficit of approximately 20% in patients who range from 1 to 10 years post TKA.[33,34] These strength deficits have been very clearly implicated in increased performance limitations (ie, walking and general mobility).[35] In our study, patients who completed the 16-week home-based exercise program demonstrated improvement in knee extensor strength of approximately 20%, consistent with previous research showing the relationship between strength and mobility resulted in significant increases in walk endurance.[36]

Our results showing improvements in strength and mobility are similar to those reported by LaStayo and colleagues,[6] who had patients perform 12 weeks of supervised resistance training in a rehabilitation clinic. Our results are particularly exciting, as the program was minimally invasive, requiring only 30 to 45 minutes 3 days per week for most patients without travel or specialized equipment. The program required only minimal supervision and feedback. This was accomplished with detailed materials and handouts and a single demonstration of the exercises, thus offering a cost-effective program to administer from a clinic.

Patients in general reported the program was enjoyable and quite easy to follow. Administration was not a significant burden on the study staff or the patients, supported by the exceptionally high compliance rates reported (nearly 80%). Previous self-reported compliance rates for home-based exercise programs is reported to be in the 50% to 60% range.[37] Patients reported the program was easily assimilated into their daily routines and this helped them stick with the program.

Although the fitness tracker technology did not appear to improve reported compliance with prescribed exercise sessions overall, patient feedback provided interesting insight that could help optimize the use of similar technology in future research. The anecdotal reports from patients who received the fitness tracker technology indicated that many participants were engaged by the device and found it motivational. This group tended to already be engaged in technology (ie, computer, and/or smart phone users), whereas those who did not favorably review the device tended to be less engaged with technology in general. Although the fitness-tracking technology is not of interest to everyone, screening to identify those who are comfortable with technology may improve the results and utility of these tools with respect to motivation and exercise programming.

Although the improvements noted in health-related and knee-related quality of life were not statistically significant, the improvements observed, especially in those with the poorest function, are encouraging and warrant further evaluation. Patient satisfaction after TKA is largely based on patient perception.[38] Failure to meet postoperative performance expectations and low 1-year WOMAC scores are among the strongest predictors of patient dissatisfaction with TKA.[38] Our home-based exercise program resulted in meaningful improvements in composite scores on the WOMAC. Future research is needed to evaluate the long-term impact these improvements might have on a patient's long-term satisfaction.

The results of this study must be interpreted with in the context of several limitations. One such limitation is the lack of a true control group to allow comparison with patients with no exercise intervention. Our study demonstrated improvement from pre-exercise to post-exercise with no overall clinical effect attributable to the fitness technology. We do not believe that these improvements are related to recovery from TKA, nor that patients would have improved without the exercise intervention; however, we could not measure that assumption. In addition, previous research does not support the idea that patients spontaneously improve after TKA but rather indicate that the deficits in normal-weight individuals who received TKA persists for many years after surgery.[12,33,35,39] Another limitation is that this study used a convenience sample recruited from an orthopedic surgery follow-up clinic and may not represent the full distribution of obese patients following TKA. In addition, patients were recruited 1 year after TKA, which did not afford the opportunity to evaluate the preoperative body habitus, functional abilities, or quality of life of the patient. We also were not able to evaluate the surgical techniques used, complications during surgery, or postoperative therapy programs, which could influence the outcomes at 1 year. Finally, our results are promising with regard to physical function and quality of life; however, the intervention was of relatively short duration, leaving the long-term durability and impact on a patient's health in question.

Longitudinal evaluations of obese patients beginning pre-TKA are needed to determine if preoperative factors are predictive of long-term functional outcomes with special attention to the role excess body weight may play. In addition, the number of obese patients receiving TKA has increased dramatically in the past decade. Systematic evaluations of postoperative rehabilitation programs may be important to understanding long-term outcomes of this growing patient population. Specifically, studies are needed on the effectiveness of the current standard programs at addressing functional recovery and durability into long-term management of TKA outcomes in obese patients. Future more comprehensive randomized clinical trials using longer duration home-based exercise intervention focused on improving the long-term functional abilities in obese individuals appear warranted based on our results.

In conclusion, obese patients receiving a TKA for debilitation OA have physical performance limitations, which remain well after patients have been released from postoperative rehabilitation. These limitations may be exacerbated by increased body weight and decreased physical activity. The combination of residual strength and conditioning deficits after TKA, low levels of physical activity, and increased physiologic and biomechanical pressure from excess body weight make these patients particularly vulnerable to poor outcome. This study provides preliminary evidence that a 16-week home-based exercise program in obese individuals 1 year post TKA is feasible and effective in improving strength and walk performance. The results of this study also indicate that a 16-week home-based exercise program may improve patient perceptions of knee function and health-related quality of life.

PRACTICAL APPLICATIONS

The article provides an in-depth evaluation of physical performance limitations, quality of life, physical activity, and patient perceptions of functional abilities in a group of older obese adults 1 year after knee replacement. Our results show that individuals have reduced physical function, low physical activity levels, and decreased quality of life after TKA. The intervention used in this study targeted these deficits in physical function after TKA with an individually tailored home-based exercise program. Our results provide valuable insight into the response to a relatively low-cost and simple-to-administer intervention, encouraging movement in patients who have completed the postoperative rehabilitation but still have physical limitations. This is among the first articles to evaluate the utility of fitness trackers in combination with prescribed exercise in older obese adults after knee replacement.

ACKNOWLEDGMENTS

The authors thank Dr Ramin Homayouni and Mr Dudley Kelso for their assistance in developing and maintaining the Redcap database, and Mrs Anita Kerkhof and Mr Tyler Ward for their assistance with subject recruitment and logistics on this project.

REFERENCES

1. Van Manen MD, Nace J, Mont MA. Management of primary knee osteoarthritis and indications for total knee arthroplasty for general practitioners. J Am Osteopath Assoc 2012;112:709–15.
2. Suri P, Morgenroth DC, Hunter DJ. Epidemiology of osteoarthritis and associated comorbidities. PM R 2012;4:S10–9.
3. Arden N, Nevitt MC. Osteoarthritis: epidemiology. Best Pract Res Clin Rheumatol 2006;20:3–25.
4. McNeil JM, Binette J. Prevalence of disabilities and associated health conditions among adults—United States. MMWR Morb Mortal Wkly Rep 1999;50:120–5.
5. Foran JRH, Mont MA, Rajadhyaksha AD, et al. Total knee arthroplasty in obese patients. J Arthroplasty 2004;19:817–24.
6. LaStayo PC, Meier W, Marcus RL, et al. Reversing muscle and mobility deficits 1 to 4 years after TKA: a pilot study. Clin Orthop Relat Res 2009;467:1493–500.
7. Bradbury N, Borton D, Spoo G, et al. Participation in sports after total knee replacement. Am J Sports Med 1998;26:530–5.
8. Aderinto J. Weight change following total hip replacement: a comparison of obese and non-obese patients. Surgeon 2005;3:269–72.
9. Heisel C, Silva M, dela Rosa MA, et al. The effects of lower-extremity total joint replacement for arthritis on obesity. Orthopedics 2005;28:157–9.
10. Unver B, Karatosun V, Bakirhan S, et al. Effects of total knee arthroplasty on body weight and functional outcome. J Phys Ther Sci 2009;21:201–6.
11. Zeni JA Jr, Snyder-Mackler L. Most patients gain weight in the 2 years after total knee arthroplasty: comparison to a healthy control group. Osteoarthritis Cartilage 2010;18:510–4.
12. Webber SC, Strachan SM, Pachu NS. Sedentary behavior, cadence, and physical activity outcomes after knee arthroplasty. Med Sci Sports Exerc 2017;49:1057–65.
13. Butler RN, Davis R, Lewis CB, et al. Physical fitness: benefits of exercise for the older patient. 2. Geriatrics 1998;53:46, 49–52, 61–2.

14. Beaupre LA, Lier D, Davies DM, et al. The effect of a preoperative exercise and education program on functional recovery, health related quality of life, and health service utilization following primary total knee arthroplasty. J Rheumatol 2004;31:1166–73.

15. Mizner RL, Petterson SC, Stevens JE, et al. Preoperative quadriceps strength predicts functional ability one year after total knee arthroplasty. J Rheumatol 2005;32:1533–9.

16. Topp R, Swank AM, Quesada PM, et al. The effect of prehabilitation exercise on strength and functioning after total knee arthroplasty. PM R 2009;1: 729–35.

17. Healy W, Iorio R, Lemos MJ. Athletic activity after total knee arthroplasty. Clin Orthop Relat Res 2000;(380):65–71.

18. Borland WS, Jennings AG. Weight loss for obese patients prior to total knee replacement. J Clin Orthop Trauma 2011;2:127–8.

19. Howarth D, Inman D, Lingard E, et al. Barriers to weight loss in obese patients with knee osteoarthritis. Ann R Coll Surg Engl 2010;92:338–40.

20. Cadmus-Bertram LA, Marcus BH, Patterson RE, et al. Randomized trial of a Fitbit-based physical activity intervention for women. Am J Prev Med 2015; 49:414–8.

21. Valbuena D, Miltenberger R, Solley E. Evaluating an Internet-based program and a behavioral coach for increasing physical activity. Behavior Analysis: Research and Practice 2015;15:122.

22. Smith W, Zucker-Levin A, Mihalko W, et al. Physical function, and physical activity in obese adults after total knee arthoplasty. Orthop Clin North Am 2017; 48(2):117–25.

23. American College of Sports Medicine, Thompson WR, Gordon NF, et al. ACSM's guidelines for exercise testing and prescription. Philadelphia: Lippincott Williams & Wilkins; 2010.

24. AmericanThroacic Society. Guidelines for the six-minute walk test. Am J Respir Crit Care Med 2002;166:111–7.

25. Enright PL, Sherrill DL. Reference equations for the six-minute walk in healthy adults. Am J Respir Crit Care Med 1998;158:1384–7.

26. Andrews AW, Thomas MW, Bohannon RW. Normative values for isometric muscle force measurements obtained with hand-held dynamometers. Phys Ther 1996;76:248–59.

27. Quintana JM, Escobar A, Arostegui I, et al. Health-related quality of life and appropriateness of knee or hip joint replacement. Arch Intern Med 2006; 166:220–6.

28. Bullens PH, van Loon CJ, de Waal Malefijt MC, et al. Patient satisfaction after total knee arthroplasty: a comparison between subjective and objective outcome assessments. J Arthroplasty 2001;16:740–7.

29. Dunbar MJ, Robertsson O, Ryd L, et al. Appropriate questionnaires for knee arthroplasty. Results of a survey of 3600 patients from the Swedish Knee Arthroplasty Registry. J Bone Joint Surg Br 2001;83: 339–44.

30. Ware JE Jr. SF-36 health survey update. Spine 2000;25:3130–9.

31. Ware JE, Snow KK, Kosinski M, et al. SF-36 health survey: manual and interpretation guide. Boston: New England Medical Center Hospital Health Institute; 1993.

32. Bohannon RW, DePasquale L. Physical Functioning Scale of the Short-Form (SF) 36: internal consistency and validity with older adults. J Geriatr Phys Ther 2010;33:16–8.

33. Berth A, Urbach D, Awiszus F. Improvement of voluntary quadriceps muscle activation after total knee arthroplasty. Arch Phys Med Rehabil 2002; 83:1432–6.

34. Huang C-H, Cheng C-K, Lee Y-T, et al. Muscle strength after successful total knee replacement: a 6- to 13-year followup. Clin Orthop Relat Res 1996;328:147–54.

35. Noble PC, Gordon MJ, Weiss JM, et al. Does total knee replacement restore normal knee function? Clin Orthop Relat Res 2005;431:157–65.

36. DiBrezzo R, Shadden BB, Raybon BH, et al. Exercise intervention designed to improve strength and dynamic balance among community-dwelling older adults. J Aging Phys Act 2005;13:198–209.

37. Linke SE, Gallo LC, Norman GJ. Attrition and adherence rates of sustained vs. intermittent exercise interventions. Ann Behav Med 2011;42: 197–209.

38. Bourne RB, Chesworth BM, Davis AM, et al. Patient satisfaction after total knee arthroplasty: who is satisfied and who is not? Clin Orthop Relat Res 2010;468:57–63.

39. Walsh M, Woodhouse LJ, Thomas SG, et al. Physical impairments and functional limitations: a comparison of individuals 1 year after total knee arthroplasty with control subjects. Phys Ther 1998; 78:248–58.

Trauma

New Imaging, Diagnostic, and Assessment Techniques in Orthopedic Trauma

Todd K. Conlan, MD[a,b], Michael J. Beebe, MD[a,b],
John C. Weinlein, MD[a,b],*

KEYWORDS

- 3D CT • O-arm • Resonant frequency analysis • Virtual stress testing • PET • Sonication • FISH
- PCR

KEY POINTS

- Three-dimensional (3D) computed tomography has improved orthopedic education and fracture interpretation.
- 3D fluoroscopy has improved intraoperative assessment of reduction and implant placement.
- Sonication, DL-dithiothreitol, and molecular techniques have improved the ability to identify infecting organisms.

INTRODUCTION

For more than a century, plain radiographs and intraoperative cultures have been the primary imaging and diagnostic modalities used in the care of orthopedic patients with injury or infection.

X-radiation, "X" representing a new and previously unknown type of radiation, was originally discovered by Wilhelm Conrad Röntgen in 1895.[1,2] The first radiograph was that of his wife's hand, who, after seeing this, declared "I have seen my death."[3] The clinical application of this new discovery quickly became apparent because its first use in a surgical operation, by John Hall-Edwards in Birmingham, United Kingdom, was only 2 months after the initial publication by Röntgen. However, Major Hall-Edwards was also one of the first to recognize the dangers of X-rays, describing X-ray dermatitis and later going on to have his arm amputated because of this same condition. Although projectional radiographs remain the staple of medical imaging, Dr William Oldendorf[4] recognized the potential for more advanced imaging using reconstruction of multiplanar radiographic imaging. His concept was used by Allan MacLeod Cormack, who later developed the mathematical basis of computed tomography (CT) scanning. Godfrey Hounsfield used these principles to develop the first commercially available CT scanner, which went into use in October 1971. Together Cormack and Hounsfield shared the 1979 Nobel Prize for Physiology or Medicine for their developments. More recently the use two-dimensional (2D) and now three-dimensional (3D) CT scans allows excellent interpretation of bony anatomy and disorder preoperatively, intraoperatively, and postoperatively.

Over the last decade and a half, similar rapid advancements in infection diagnosis have changed the perioperative evaluation of patients. From the first cultures of *Bacillus anthracis* by Robert Koch in 1876, clinicians have progressed the knowledge of culture mediums and stains specific to various bacterial causes. However, the culture methods established in the late 1800s[5] have generally remained

[a] University of Tennessee-Campbell Clinic, Department of Orthopaedic Surgery and Biomedical Engineering, 1211 Union Avenue, Suite 500, Memphis, TN 38117, USA; [b] Regional One Health, 877 Jefferson Avenue, Memphis, TN 38103, USA
* Corresponding author. 1211 Union Avenue, Suite 500, Memphis, TN 38117.
E-mail address: jweinlein@campbellclinic.com

Orthop Clin N Am 50 (2019) 47–56
https://doi.org/10.1016/j.ocl.2018.08.010
0030-5898/19/© 2018 Elsevier Inc. All rights reserved.

unchanged in that they still have time constraints as well as varying, sometimes unacceptable, sensitivity and specificity depending on the bacteria and culture medium.[6] New technology has focused on increasing the sensitivity, specificity, and time to identification of bacteria, leading to improved patient care and eradication of operative infections.

This article examines new imaging, diagnostic, and assessment techniques that may have great impact on the care of patients with orthopedic trauma with injury and/or infection.

EDUCATION AND FRACTURE INTERPRETATION

Three-dimensional reconstruction of CT scans has the potential to enhance preoperative planning and surgical education. Although consideration of radiation exposure with CT scanning is important, reconstructing acquired data into 3 dimensions does not increase radiation dose, but it provides the ability to better facilitate education for medical students and residents and improves the learning curve for young orthopedic surgeons. The same technology is also used in computer-assisted surgery (CAS), allowing surgeons to develop forward planning, awareness of problems, flexible decision making, and mental readiness.[7]

Owing to their complex 3D anatomy and fracture morphology, acetabular and pelvic ring fractures are difficult to treat and are associated with a steep learning curve. The use of 3D CT scan reconstructions preoperatively with the combination of standard plain films and CT reconstructed 2D images has been shown to quicken the learning curve for inexperienced orthopedic surgeons.[8] Semiautomatic segmentation, the process of separating acetabular fracture fragments by color, was used in the training of orthopedic residents on the classification of acetabular fractures. Excellent overall intraclass correlation coefficient (ICC) = 0.88,[9] a measure of how similarly participants in a group answer, was seen and acetabular classification accuracy improved. Computer models of the 3D reconstructed pelvis have shown promise in small series when integrated with haptic feedback, creating the sense of touch through vibrational forces, to allow surgeons to reconstruct the fracture preoperatively.[10,11] In addition, 3D printing of a patient's pelvis allows preoperative bending of plates and in a small clinical series showed reduction of operating room (OR) time and blood loss with improved reduction.[12] No large clinical series currently exist regarding

CAS in preoperative planning, although its future use seems promising.

Proximal humerus fractures represent another area of the body where complex fractures lead to disagreements about fracture patterns and treatment plans. Studies examining the use of 3D and 2D reconstruction CT scans of the proximal humerus have been mixed, with lack of interobserver agreement among fully trained orthopedic and trauma surgeons.[13] Similar to acetabular fractures, the use of 3D CT scans does not add to the interobserver or intraobserver agreement between experienced surgeons, but does aid to diminish the learning curve among evaluators with limited clinical experience.[14]

Three-dimensional reconstruction imaging has proved to be a valuable tool in the understanding of fracture morphology in complex periarticular injury. In looking at Hoffa fractures of the distal femur, recreating a 3D map of the reconstructed fracture allowed analysis of location and frequency of fracture lines and areas of comminution.[15] Three-dimensional reconstruction has also been applied to calcaneus fractures delineating the fracture morphology of tongue-type calcaneal fractures and appropriateness of percutaneous fixation and reduction maneuvers.[16]

Using CT scans has also had an impact in the immediate work-up of patients with polytrauma. CT scan has 100% sensitivity in detecting traumatic knee arthrotomies compared with 92% sensitivity for the saline load test.[17] CT angiography can offer a quicker and less morbid evaluation of potential extremity vascular injuries (ankle-brachial index [ABI]<0.9), showing 100% sensitivity and specificity for vascular injury compared with the gold standard conventional arteriography; significant cost savings can also be obtained.[18] Although CT angiography is highly sensitive, specific, and cost-effective, clinicians must still be judicious in its application and avoid using it in patients without risk factors for vascular injury in the setting of normal pulses.[19]

FRACTURE TREATMENT
Three-Dimensional Fluoroscopy

Fluoroscopy has had a monumental role in the ability of surgeons to treat fractures in the operative theater. As preoperative surgical imaging has increased to use both 2D and 3D reconstruction CT, the need for intraoperative CT reconstructed imaging in complex periarticular, pelvic, and acetabular fractures has become necessary. Three second-generation mobile 3D C-arm models currently exist: the Ziehm Vision

FD Vario 3D and Ziehm Vision RFD 3D imaging system (Ziehm Imaging, Nürnberg, Germany) and the ARCADIS 3D (Siemens, Erlangen, Germany).

The Ziehm Vision FD Vario 3D, which replaced the previous Ziehm Vario 3D, has an isocentric design that requires only a 135° arc of motion obtaining 100 fluoroscopic images in 1 minute for a scan. Each scan has a 3D volume size of $12.8 \times 12.8 \times 12.8$ cm, $256^3/512^3$ voxel. The larger Ziehm Vision RFD 3D is more suitable for pelvic surgery with a larger 3D volume size of $19.8 \times 19.6 \times 18.0$ cm, $320^3/512^3$ voxel. This isocentric design requires a 180° arc of motion and 3 minutes to complete a scan. The Ziehm Vision RFD 3D cost is estimated at US$68,000 more than a conventional C-arm. The ARCADIS Orbic 3D, which replaced the Siremobil Iso-C 3D, uses a 190° unstopped arc of motion to collect 100 fluoroscopic images, requiring 3 minutes to complete a scan. The 3D volume size is $12 \times 12 \times 12$ cm. Siemens proprietary 3D integration allows visualization of preoperatively obtained MRI with intraoperative CT. Both companies allow open-source compatibility with leading manufacturing navigation systems in addition to their own proprietary software. In addition, both can be used reliably as 2D C-arms. Studies of the first-generation models, ISO-C 3D and Vario 3D, showed superiority of the ISO-C 3D in visualizing joint surfaces. However, the Vario 3D, because of its arc of motion, proved superior in shoulder surgery and patients with morbid obesity.[20] It was noted in this study that image quality of both mobile 3D C-arms was adequate to make clinical decisions.

In contrast with the motorized mobile C-arm, the O-arm intraoperative CT system (Medtronic Navigation, Louisville, CO) has 3D and 2D capabilities but is more cumbersome to work around while using it as a 2D C-arm. The O-arm offers a larger field of view (39.70 cm $\times$ 15 cm) compared with mobile C-arms; however, the O-arm is much larger (925.8 kg) and has a higher cost, estimated at US$900,000. The O-arm uses a 360° arc of motion to collect 745 images. The O-arm does not support nonproprietary navigation. Radiation levels are higher than those of mobile 3D C-arms; however, in evaluating radiation exposure from 1 scan of the thoracic spine using the O-arm, dosages were less than those of a conventional CT scan. At a distance greater than 2 m from the isocenter of the O-arm, dosage was minimal at 11 ± 1 μSv.[21]

Cost savings of these systems are achieved through prevention of the need to return to the OR for malpositioned implants or unsatisfactory reduction, often detected only by postoperative CT scan. ISO-C 3D images have been found to be equivalent to postoperative CT scan.[22] Over a 5-year period in a study of routine use of postoperative pelvic CT in the setting of percutaneous pelvic fixation using standard 2D fluoroscopy, the investigators found a 6% (10 patients) revision rate. Postoperative anteroposterior radiographs had 27% sensitivity for detecting malpositioned implants.[23] Most alarming in this study was that, in patients deemed to have safe implants on perioperative imaging, 4% (7 out of 148) eventually required revision surgery because of malposition of implants.

However, in the foot and ankle literature, Iso-C 3D imaging has not been shown to decrease the malreduction in operatively treated syndesmosis injuries compared with standard fluoroscopy.[24] 3D imaging intraoperatively does have a small increase in operative time caused by the length of the scan. The average time for acquisition and evaluation for ISO-C 3D and ARCADIS-3D was 330 and 240 seconds respectively. Thirty-nine percent of ISO-C 3D and 34% of ARCADIS-3D (24 and 21) cases had a change in reduction or implant position after scan.[25] Another study in distal radius fractures showed an additional 6.7 minutes of operative time when using the ARCADIS-3D but with a change in screw placement caused by recognized malposition in 31.3% of surgeries.[26] In posterior wall acetabular fractures, 1 small series showed that ISO-C 3D imaging revealed instability in 1 of 5 fractures that was initially found to be stable with standard fluoroscopy necessitating surgical fixation.[27] Three-dimensional imaging can confirm reduction before leaving the OR in management of posterior sternoclavicular dislocation, reductions that are difficult to visualize using 2D imaging.[28] The limitation of most of these studies is lack of clinical outcomes in relation to reduction and implant placement; further study is warranted.

COMPUTED TOMOGRAPHY–GUIDED NAVIGATION

In addition to preventing return to the OR because of misplacement of surgical implants, 3D intraoperative imaging offers the capabilities to work with CAS. The goals of CAS are to reduce surgical time and radiation exposure while increasing accuracy during placement of implants. The use of navigation is well documented in the spine surgery literature; it has been in use since 1995[29] for more accurate placement of pedicle screws. Multiple studies have shown reduction of pedicle breaches from 6% to 30% using conventional fluoroscopy[30–32] to 5% with 3D guided navigation.[33,34]

More recently, navigation in the pelvis has been reported with conflicting results. A study out of the Netherlands found increased need for reoperation caused by malposition of implants in the CAS group compared with traditional fluoroscopy, although the study was underpowered and the results did not meet clinical significance.[35] Smaller series have shown that 3D navigation can reduce OR time, radiation exposure, and blood loss in placement of retrograde anterior column screws[36] as well as safe placement of iliosacral screws.[37] Navigation depends on intraoperative 3D imaging and registering of instrumentation in space. Navigation is only as good as the registration of data; any change to the position of the patient after registration or position of the optical tracking instruments in space could result in potential misplacement of implants. Further clinical studies are needed in the pelvis and acetabulum to establish safety of CT-navigated surgery in comparison with traditional techniques.

ASSESSMENT OF UNION

Orthopedic Surgeons use subjective measures to assess bone healing. Typical assessment involves observing callus formation on radiographs and clinical assessment determining pain with ambulation and tenderness with palpation at the fracture site.[38] A cross-sectional survey of 577 orthopedic surgeons revealed no consensus regarding the assessment of union in tibia fractures.[39]

RADIOGRAPHIC UNION SCORE FOR HIP/ RADIOGRAPHIC UNION SCORE FOR TIBIA

In an attempt to make the assessment of union more objective the RUSH (radiographic union score for hip) and RUST (radiographic union score for tibia) scores were created based on orthogonal plain radiographs. The RUSH score involves evaluating and grading cortical bridging, disappearance of cortical fracture line, amount of trabecular consolidation, and disappearance of trabecular fracture line. Agreement improved significantly between radiologists and orthopedic surgeons with the adaptation of the RUSH (ICC = 0.85 and 0.88 in femoral neck and intertrochanteric femur fractures respectively).[40,41] RUST involves evaluation of 4 cortices of the diaphyseal tibia and scoring the presence of callus and visibility of fracture line. Similar ICC was observed

with the RUST.[42,43] The modified RUST was created to address metaphyseal fractures,[44] the modified score delineates whether callus is present or bridging. ICC was higher than the standard RUST for metaphyseal fractures using this modified criterion.

RESONANT FREQUENCY ANALYSIS

Resonant frequency analysis (RFA) of bone allows the evaluation of its stiffness to be observed objectively as it heals. RFA is obtained by an impulse frequency response, a brief tap on the tibia that is then recorded by an accelerometer.[45] The average is then compared with the uninjured side to give a tibial stiffness index. RFA was found to be useful in fractures without fixation and fractures treated with unlocked, unreamed tibial nails and external fixators. RFA was not useful in locked reamed tibial nails. New interest in RFA has been applied through excitation of external fixator pins with promising results[46,47]; however, further validation in clinical series is necessary.

VIRTUAL STRESS TESTING

Virtual stress testing takes a patient's CT scan of healing bone and incorporates it into a finite element modeling. This noninvasive bone strength assessment tool was applied retrospectively in a case series of patients who were treated for open comminuted tibia fractures with circular fixators in a military population.[48] CT data were analyzed through a series of computer models that tested the bone to failure through simulated compression and torsional loads. This technology is promising and may provide an objective measure of when to begin weight bearing in this complex patient population.

18F-PET/MRI

First established in 2010, ^{18}F-fluoride PET/MRI is a combination of the soft tissue imaging of MRI with the metabolic activity of a PET scan.[49] PET/MRI is just beginning to be used for nononcologic musculoskeletal diseases. In a small clinical series, patients with negative radiographs were diagnosed with stress reactions after undergoing 18F-PET/MRI.[50] PET/MRI is promising but still limited by clinical availability and reimbursement.

SEROLOGIC MARKERS FOR BONE UNION

Serologic markers are an exciting developing field in assessment of bone union, having previously been used in osteoporosis.[51] Tartrate-resistant acid phosphatase 5b and C-terminal cross-linking telopeptide of type I collagen, both markers of osteoclast activity, were shown retrospectively to be associated with fracture union.[52] Collagen III amino-terminal propeptide, a marker for early callus formation, was higher during the first 10 weeks in patients going on to nonunion.[53] Collagen I carboxy-terminal propeptide and bone-specific alkaline phosphatase, both markers of osteo-blast activity, were decreased after 10 weeks in the same study.[53] Serologic markers are compli-cated by the variability of values between pa-tients and at this time are still experimental.[54]

PET AND PET/CT

Infection is a significant complication after fracture treatment. Infection is consistently asso-ciated with fracture nonunion. Treatment recom-mendations and outcomes for nonunions vary considerably based on the presence or absence of infection. Traditional nuclear medicine scan-ning, although helpful in some areas of ortho-pedics, has not been consistently useful in the diagnosis of infection associated with nonunion.[55,56] Stucken and colleagues[56] evalu-ated the usefulness of nuclear medicine scanning (indium-111–labeled white blood cell [WBC] scanning, technetium-99m scintigraphy, or com-bined indium-111/technetium-99m scintigraphy) in the preoperative evaluation of fracture nonunion. The sensitivity of nuclear medicine scanning in this study was only 19%. When using results of nuclear medicine scanning with WBC count, C-reactive protein (CRP), and erythrocyte sedimentation rate (ESR) for predictive value of infection, 3 positive tests resulted in a positive predictive value for infection of 85.7%. When nu-clear scanning was not used (leaving WBC count, CRP, and ESR), 3 positive tests resulted in a pos-itive predictive value of 100%.

PET and combined PET/CT are being used with increased frequency outside the United States in the detection of infection.[57–59] An early meta-analysis suggested that PET has the high-est sensitivity (96%) and specificity (91%) compared with bone scintigraphy, leukocyte scintigraphy, combined bone/leukocyte scintig-raphy, and MRI in the diagnosis of chronic oste-omyelitis.[60] CT added to PET increases specificity.[61] CT adds anatomic information rele-vant for characterization and treatment of infection.[62]

PET is based on fluorodeoxyglucose (FDG), a radiolabeled glucose analogue that is easily taken up by macrophages, neutrophils, and lym-phocytes. This uptake may be the reason PET is helpful in chronic infections in which macro-phages predominate.[63] Shemesh and col-leagues[57] reported the results of a small series of tibial implant–related infections (n = 10) using PET/CT. Sensitivity was 85.7%, whereas speci-ficity was 100%. Positive tests were based on up-take at the bone/prosthesis interface because some clinicians believe the uptake at the bone/prosthesis interface is the best indicator of implant-related infection.[61] vanVliet and col-leagues[59] in a larger series (n = 30) reported on the utility of PET/CT in the evaluation of lower extremity delayed unions. The investiga-tors used a more quantitative approach to the diagnosis of infection using the maximum stan-dardized uptake value (SUV_{max}) of FDG. SUV_{max} was greater in patients with infected delayed unions than aseptic delayed unions. When an SUV_{max} cutoff value of 4.0 was used, the sensi-tivity and specificity were 65% and 77% respec-tively. Wenter and colleagues[58] reported a sensitivity and specificity of 83% and 89% respectively when considering PET/CT for the diagnosis of implant-related infection. These in-vestigators used both quantitative and semi-quantitative methods in determining presence of infection.

One advantage of PET or PET/CT is time. PET results are generally available in 1 to 3 hours[57,63] and PET using quantitative analysis can be done quicker than semiquantitative analysis.[58] Lack of a standardized diagnostic criterion remains an issue for PET and PET/CT.[58] Another issue with PET and PET/CT involves the short half-life of FDG. Because of this short half-life, facilities within the hospital are necessary to process FDG and this in-house processing must be a consideration in cost.[6] Further investigation is necessary to determine whether PET/CT has a role in the diagnosis of implant-related infection and infection associated with nonunion.

ORGANISM IDENTIFICATION

Diagnosis of infection in orthopedics has tradi-tionally been based on intraoperative cultures. Intraoperative tissue cultures have been shown to have higher sensitivity (93% vs 70%) than intraoperative swabs in evaluation of peripros-thetic joint infection.[64] The sensitivity of culture methods for detection of pathogens associated with nonunions seems significantly worse compared with molecular techniques.[65]

The techniques for processing cultures remain largely unchanged since the late 1800s.[6] These techniques involve the ability of free-floating bacteria to grow on agar. However, bacteria that are not free floating and have created a biofilm do not grow with traditional techniques. Although optimizing the collection and transport of a specimen may increase the yield of free-floating bacteria, this optimization likely does not help with bacteria in biofilms.

SONICATION

Sonication is a technique of improving culture sensitivity by driving bacteria out of biofilms. Sonication can only be done after implant removal. Sonication involves the utilization of ultrasound to disaggregate biofilms.[6] Sonication has been shown to improve sensitivity and specificity of tissue culture associated with removal of spinal implants.[66] Sensitivity and specificity were 91% and 97% with sonication, respectively, versus 73% and 93% without sonication. Similar results were shown with sonication after intramedullary nail removal. Esteban and colleagues[67] reported the results of sonication after removal of 31 intramedullary nails. Eight out of 31 cases had preoperative clinical signs of infection (ie, purulence). Other common reasons for nail removal included nonunion and pain. Cultures of 15 out of 31 nails were positive after sonication. Note that patients with pain and positive cultures after sonication improved with nail removal. Although sonication seems to improve sensitivity of tissue culture, implant removal is necessary. Clinical situations exist in which union can be obtained if there are positive intraoperative cultures while maintaining implants. Berkes and colleagues[68] reported a 71% incidence of union after early postoperative infection with debridement, maintenance of implants, and suppression to union with culture-specific antibiotics.

DL-Dithiothreitol

DL-Dithiothreitol (DTT) is a chemical debonding technique that also has the goal of driving bacteria out of biofilms. A potential advantage of DTT compared with sonication is that tissue can also be evaluated without implants.[69] Drago and colleagues[70] compared DTT with sonication in 76 patients with prosthetic joint infection or aseptic loosening. Sensitivity was better with DTT (85.7%) versus sonication (71.4%), whereas both had identical specificity (94.1%). DTT had better sensitivity and specificity compared with standard tissue culture. A recent study supports the potential cost benefits of both DTT and sonication compared with standard culture.[71]

Molecular Techniques
Fluorescence in situ hybridization
Fluorescence in situ hybridization (FISH) is a technique that uses fluorescent labeled 16S ribosomal RNA (rRNA) and 23S rRNA probes that have been engineered to target specific bacteria.[65,72,73] Confocal laser scanning microscopy is then used to directly visualize bacteria. FISH is limited by having to determine a priori which microorganisms are being sought. An organism not specifically being sought with an appropriate probe cannot be identified. FISH has the ability to confirm the presence of specific microorganisms but has no role in the identification of new or novel microorganisms. FISH is often used to validate other techniques.

Polymerase chain reaction
Polymerase chain reaction (PCR) is a technique that allows amplification of bacterial DNA or RNA. Nucleic acids present in a sample are first extracted and then amplified through the use of primers. Primers with nucleic acid sequences unique to 16S ribosomal DNA are often used. Other gene sequences can also be used.[74,75] Single-primer PCR is limited in that only 1 organism can be identified.[65] Analysis begins once amplification and the generation of amplicons are complete.

One method of analysis is weighing the amplicons with mass spectrometry to determine base composition. This base composition allows identification of bacteria. The PLEX-ID System (Abbott Ibis Biosciences) is a PCR/electrospray ionization mass spectrometry (ESI-MS) system. All organisms comprising greater than 1% of the local microbial population are identified.[74,75] Results are available between 60 minutes and 8 hours. Results using this technique for identification of pathogens in septic arthritis and osteoarthritis were recently reported.[76] PCR/ESI-MS identified microorganisms in 50% of cases of suspected septic arthritis compared with 16% of cases with standard culture techniques. This same system was studied in the evaluation of nonunions. Thirty-four nonunions were assessed using PCR/ESI-MS and standard culture techniques. Cultures were positive in only 8 cases, whereas PCR/ESI-MS identified microorganisms in 30 cases. FISH confirmed the findings of PCR/ESI-MS. PCR/ESI-MS identified multiple organisms in 62% of cases.[62]

The US Food and Drug Administration has approved several multiplex PCR systems for clinical application, although none are currently orthopedic specific.[77] BioFire is one such company that has panels available in 4 different areas (respiratory, blood, gastrointestinal, meningitis/encephalitis).[78] Results are reported to be available in approximately 1 hour. Multiplex panels have shown high sensitivity in the detection of gastrointestinal pathogens.[79] A panel of common organisms responsible for orthopedic infections with results available in 1 hour could be useful.

PCR is also being used in the identification of patients with methicillin-resistant *Staphylococcus aureus* (MRSA) nasal colonization. A large randomized controlled trial of surgical patients with MRSA nasal colonization treated with mupirocin ointment and chlorhexidine gluconate soap resulted in an overall *Staphylococcus* infection rate of 3.4% (vs 7.7% in the placebo group). The rate of deep surgical site infection was 0.9% in the treatment group (vs 4.4% in the placebo group).[80] Rapid identification of MRSA is extremely important in the trauma population if timely treatment is to be initiated.

SEROLOGIC MARKERS FOR INFECTION

Local biomarkers (synovial biomarkers) have been discussed in the detection of prosthetic joint infection. The presence of leukocyte esterase in synovial fluid after total joint arthroplasty has shown sensitivity and specificity of 81% to 93% and 97% respectively for the diagnosis of infection.[81,82] This test is inexpensive to administer, costing approximately $0.17 per test. The results of this test are also available very quickly.[83] This cost differentiates this biomarker from others that may have better sensitivity. Alpha defensin is a peptide secreted by host neutrophils in response to the presence of a pathogen. The presence of synovial alpha defensin has shown sensitivity and specificity of 100% and 96% respectively.[81] Alpha defensin is not affected by prior antibiotic use but may be affected by metallosis.[84] This test has been costly in the past and at some institutions[83]; however, this cost seems to be decreasing.[85] These tests seem to be valuable in the detection of infection after total joint arthroplasty. What remains to be seen is whether any of these local biomarkers are relevant to the diagnosis of infection after fracture fixation. Some practitioners routinely include aspiration for culture in the work-up of nonunion.[86] The sensitivity and specificity of aspirating and culturing fluid around a nonunion, to our knowledge, is not known. Perhaps the presence of local biomarkers at the site of fracture or nonunion will lead to improvement in the diagnosis of infection.

SUMMARY

Imaging, diagnostic testing, and assessment techniques in orthopedic trauma continue to advance rapidly. Three-dimensional imaging has assisted in fracture assessment preoperatively, whereas improvement in C-arm technology has allowed real-time evaluation of implant placement and periarticular reduction by surgeons before leaving the OR. Similarly, advances in imaging techniques have allowed earlier and more accurate diagnosis of nonunion and infection. Innovations in bacteriologic testing have led to improvement in the sensitivity and specificity of perioperative and peri-implant infections, which has improved the care that surgeons provide to their patients. As medical technology continues to improve, it is critical that surgeons remain up to date on the options available for optimal patient care.

REFERENCES

1. Rontgen WC. On a new kind of rays. Science 1896; 3:227–31.
2. International Society for Computed Tomography. Available at: http://www.isct.org. Accessed July 22, 2018.
3. Landwehr G. Wilhelm Conrad Röntgen and the beginning of modern physics. In: Haase A, Landwehr G, Umbach E, editors. Röntgen Centennial. X-rays in Natural and Life Sciences. Singapore: World Scientific Publishing; 1997. p. 7–8. ISBN 981-02-3085-0.
4. Oldendorf WH. Isolated flying spot detection of radiodensity discontinuities – displaying the internal structural pattern of a complex object. Ire Trans Biomed Electron 1961;BME-8:68–72.
5. Koch R. An address on cholera and its bacillus. Br Med J 1884;2:453–9.
6. Firoozabadi R, Alton T, Wenke J. Novel strategies for the diagnosis of posttraumatic infections in orthopaedic trauma patients. J Am Acad Orthop Surg 2015;23:443–51.
7. Boudissa M, Courvoisier A, Chabanas M, et al. Computer assisted surgery in preoperative planning of acetabular fracture surgery: state of the art. Expert Rev Med Devices 2018;15(1):81–9.
8. Jouffroy P, Sebaaly A, Aubert T, et al. Improved acetabular fracture diagnosis after training in a CT-based method. Orthop Traumatol Surg Res 2017;103(3):325–9.
9. Boudissa M, Orfeuvre B, Chabanas M, et al. Does semi-automatic bone-fragment segmentation improve the reproducibility of the Letournel acetabular fracture classification? Orthop Traumatol Surg Res 2017;103(5):633–8.

10. Kovler I, Joskowicz L, Weil YA, et al. Haptic computer-assisted patient-specific preoperative planning for orthopedic fractures surgery. Int J Comput Assist Radiol Surg 2015;10(10):1535–46.

11. Fornaro J, Keel M, Harders M, et al. An interactive surgical planning tool for acetabular fractures: initial results. J Orthop Surg Res 2010;5:50.

12. Maini L, Sharma A, Jha S, et al. Three-dimensional printing and patient-specific pre-contoured plate: future of acetabulum fracture fixation? Eur J Trauma Emerg Surg 2018;44(2):215–24.

13. Bruinsma WE, Guitton TG, Warner JJ, et al. Interobserver reliability of classification and characterization of proximal humeral fractures: a comparison of two and three-dimensional CT. J Bone Joint Surg Am 2013;95(17):1600–4.

14. Berkes MB, Dines JS, Little MT, et al. The impact of three-dimensional CT imaging on intraobserver and interobserver reliability of proximal humeral fracture classifications and treatment recommendations. J Bone Joint Surg Am 2014;96(15):1281–6.

15. Xie X, Zhan Y, Dong M, et al. Two and three-dimensional CT mapping of Hoffa fractures. J Bone Joint Surg Am 2017;99(21):1866–74.

16. Mitchell PM, O'Neill DE, Gallagher B, et al. Pathoanatomy of the tongue-type calcaneus fracture: assessment using 2- and 3-dimensional computed tomography. J Orthop Trauma 2018;32(5):e161–5.

17. Konda SR, Davidovitch RI, Egol KA. Computed tomography scan to detect traumatic arthrotomies and identify periarticular wounds not requiring surgical intervention: an improvement over the saline load test. J Orthop Trauma 2013;27(9):498–504.

18. Seamon MJ, Smoger D, Torres DM, et al. A prospective validation of a current practice: the detection of extremity vascular injury with CT angiography. J Trauma 2009;67(2):238–43.

19. Monazzam S, Goodell PB, Salcedo ES, et al. When are CT angiograms indicated for patients with lower extremity fractures? A review of 275 extremities. J Trauma Acute Care Surg 2017;82(1):133–7.

20. Stübig T, Kendoff D, Citak M, et al. Comparative study of different intraoperative 3-D image intensifiers in orthopedic trauma care. J Trauma 2009;66(3):821–30.

21. Pitteloud N, Gamulin A, Barea C, et al. Radiation exposure using the O-arm surgical imaging system. Eur Spine J 2017;26(3):651–7.

22. Hott JS, Papadopoulos SM, Theodore N, et al. Intraoperative Iso-C C-arm navigation in cervical spinal surgery: review of the first 52 cases. Spine 2004;29(24):2856.

23. Elnahal WA, Vetharajan N, Mohamed B, et al. Routine postoperative computed tomography scans after pelvic fracture fixation: a necessity or a luxury? J Orthop Trauma 2018;32(Suppl 1): S66–71.

24. Davidovitch RI, Weil Y, Karia R, et al. Intraoperative syndesmotic reduction: three-dimensional versus standard fluoroscopic imaging. J Bone Joint Surg Am 2013;95(20):1838–43.

25. Richter M, Zech S. Intraoperative 3-dimensional imaging in foot and ankle trauma-experience with a second-generation device (ARCADIS-3D). J Orthop Trauma 2009;23(3):213–20.

26. Mehling I, Rittstieg P, Mehling AP, et al. Intraoperative C-arm CT imaging in angular stable plate osteosynthesis of distal radius fractures. J Hand Surg Eur 2013;38(7):751–7.

27. Cunningham B, Jackson K, Ortega G. Intraoperative CT in the assessment of posterior wall acetabular fracture stability. Orthopedics 2014; 37(4):e328–31.

28. Sullivan JP, Warme BA, Wolf BR. Use of an O-arm intraoperative computed tomography scanner for closed reduction of posterior sternoclavicular dislocations. J Shoulder Elbow Surg 2012;21(3):e17–20.

29. Rahmathulla G, Nottmeier EW, Pirris SM, et al. Intraoperative image-guided spinal navigation: technical pitfalls and their avoidance. Neurosurg Focus 2014;36(3):E3.

30. Abumi K, Shono Y, Ito M, et al. Complications of pedicle screw fixation in reconstructive surgery of the cervical spine. Spine 2000;25(8):962–9.

31. Heary RF, Bono CM, Black M. Thoracic pedicle screws: postoperative computerized tomography scanning assessment. J Neurosurg 2004;100(4 Suppl Spine):325–31.

32. Kosmopoulos V, Schizas C. Pedicle screw placement accuracy: a meta-analysis. Spine 2007;32(3): E111–20.

33. Hott JS, Deshmukh VR, Klopfenstein JD, et al. Intraoperative Iso-C C-arm navigation in craniospinal surgery: the first 60 cases. Neurosurgery 2004; 54(5):1131–6.

34. Ito Y, Sugimoto Y, Tomioka M, et al. Clinical accuracy of 3D fluoroscopy-assisted cervical pedicle screw insertion. J Neurosurg Spine 2008;9(5):450–3.

35. Verbeek J, Hermans E, van Vugt A, et al. Correct positioning of percutaneous iliosacral screws with computer-navigated versus fluoroscopically guided surgery in traumatic pelvic ring fractures. J Orthop Trauma 2016;30(6):331–5.

36. He J, Tan G, Zhou D, et al. Comparison of isocentric C-arm 3-dimensional navigation and conventional fluoroscopy for percutaneous retrograde screwing for anterior column fracture of acetabulum: an observational study. Medicine (Baltimore) 2016;95(2):e2470.

37. Coste C, Asloum Y, Marcheix PS, et al. Percutaneous iliosacral screw fixation in unstable pelvic ring lesions: the interest of O-ARM CT-guided navigation. Orthop Traumatol Surg Res 2013;99(4 Suppl):S273–8.

38. Cunningham BP, Brazina S, Morshed S, et al. Fracture healing: a review of clinical, imaging and laboratory diagnostic options. Injury 2017;48(Suppl 1): S69–75.

39. Bhandari M, Guyatt GH, Swiontkowski MF, et al. A lack of consensus in the assessment of fracture healing among orthopedic surgeons. J Orthop Trauma 2002;16(8):562–6.

40. Bhandari M, Chiavaras MM, Parasu N, et al. Radiographic union score for hip substantially improves agreement between surgeons and radiologists. BMC Musculoskelet Disord 2013;14:70.

41. Chiavaras MM, Bains S, Choudur H, et al. The Radiographic Union Score for Hip (RUSH): the use of a checklist to evaluate hip fracture healing improves agreement between radiologists and orthopedic surgeons. Skeletal Radiol 2013;42(8):1079–88.

42. Whelan DB, Bhandari M, Stephen D, et al. Development of the radiographic union score for tibial fractures for the assessment of tibial fracture healing after intramedullary fixation. J Trauma 2010;68(3): 629–32.

43. Whelan DB, Bhandari M, McKee MD, et al. Interobserver and intraobserver variation in the assessment of the healing of tibial fractures after intramedullary fixation. J Bone Joint Surg Br 2002; 84(1):15–8.

44. Litrenta J, Tornetta P, Mehta S, et al. Determination of radiographic healing: an assessment of consistency using RUST and modified RUST in metadiaphyseal fractures. J Orthop Trauma 2015;29(11): 516–20.

45. Tower SS, Beals RK, Duwelius PJ. Resonant frequency analysis of the tibia as a measure of fracture healing. J Orthop Trauma 1993;7(6):552–7.

46. Mattei L, Longo A, Di Puccio F, et al. Vibration testing procedures for bone stiffness assessment in fractures treated with external fixation. Ann Biomed Eng 2017;45(4):1111–21.

47. Mattei L, Di Puccio F, Marchetti S. In vivo impact testing on a lengthened femur with external fixation: a future option for the non-invasive monitoring of fracture healing? J R Soc Interface 2018; 15(142) [pii:20180068].

48. Petfield JL, Hayeck GT, Kopperdahl DL, et al. Virtual stress testing of fracture stability in soldiers with severely comminuted tibial fractures. J Orthop Res 2017;35(4):805–11.

49. Kogan F, Broski SM, Yoon D, et al. Applications of PET-MRI in musculoskeletal disease. J Magn Reson Imaging 2018;48(1):27–47.

50. Crönlein M, Rauscher I, Beer AJ, et al. Visualization of stress fractures of the foot using PET-MRI: a feasibility study. Eur J Med Res 2015;20:99.

51. Cox G, Einhorn TA, Tzioupis C, et al. Bone-turnover markers in fracture healing. J Bone Joint Surg Br 2010;92(3):329–34.

52. Moghaddam A, Müller U, Roth HJ, et al. TRACP 5b and CTX as osteological markers of delayed fracture healing. Injury 2011;42(8):758–64.

53. Kurdy NM. Serology of abnormal fracture healing: the role of PIIINP, PICP, and BsALP. J Orthop Trauma 2000;14(1):48–53.

54. Pountos I, Georgouli T, Pneumaticos S, et al. Fracture non-union: can biomarkers predict outcome? Injury 2013;44(12):1725–32.

55. Jarmon N, Sirkin MS, Kinchelow T. Utility of white blood cell scanning in detecting infections associated with nonunions. Presented as a podium exhibit at the 76th Annual Meeting of the American Academy of Orthopaedic Surgeons; 2009 Feb 25-28; Las Vegas, NV. Paper #178.

56. Stucken C, Olszewski DC, Creevy WR, et al. Preoperative diagnosis of infection in patients with nonunions. J Bone Joint Surg Am 2013;95:1409.

57. Shemesh S, Kosashvili Y, Groshar D, et al. The value of 18-FDG PET/CT in the diagnosis and management of implant-related infections of the tibia: a case series. Injury 2016;45:1377–82.

58. Wenter V, Muller J, Alber NL, et al. The diagnostic value of 18F FDG PET for the detection of chronic osteomyelitis and implant-associated. Eur J Nucl Med Mol Imaging 2016;34:749–61.

59. vanVliet KE, de Jong VM, Termaat, et al. FDG-PET/CT for differentiating between aseptic and septic delayed union in the lower extremity. Arch Orthop Trauma Surg 2018;138:189–94.

60. Termaat MF, Raijmakers PG, Scholten HJ, et al. The accuracy of diagnostic imaging for the assessment of chronic osteomyelitis: a systematic review and meta-analysis. J Bone Joint Surg Am 2005;11: 2464–71.

61. van der Bruggen W, Bleeker-Rovers CP, Boerman OC, et al. PET and SPECT in osteomyelitis and prosthetic bone and joint infections: a systematic review. Semin Nucl Med 2010;40: 3–15.

62. Hartmann A, Eid K, Dora C, et al. Diagnostic value of 18F-FDG PET/CT in trauma patients with suspected chronic osteomyelitis. Eur J Nucl Med Mol Imaging 2007;34:704–14.

63. Stumpe KDM, Strobel K. 18F FDG-PET imaging in musculoskeletal infection. Q J Nucl Med Mol Imaging 2006;50:131–42.

64. Aggarwal VK, Higuera C, Deirmengian G, et al. Swab cultures are not as effective as tissue cultures for diagnosis of periprosthetic joint infection. Clin Orthop Relat Res 2013;471:3196–203.

65. Palmer MP, Altman DT, Altman GT, et al. Can we trust intraoperative culture results in nonunions? J Orthop Trauma 2014;28:384–90.

66. Sampedro MF, Huddleston PM, Piper KE, et al. A biofilm approach to detect bacteria on removed spinal implants. Spine 2010;35:1218–24.

67. Esteban J, Sandoval E, Cordero-Ampuero J, et al. Sonication of intramedullary nails: clinically-related infection and contamination. Open Orthop J 2012;6:255–60.

68. Berkes M, Obremskey WT, Scannell B, et al. Maintenance of hardware after early postoperative infection following fracture internal fixation. J Bone Joint Surg Am 2010;92:823–8.

69. De Vecci E, Bottagisio M, Bortolin M, et al. Improving the bacterial recovery by using dithiothreitol with aerobic and anaerobic broth in biofilm-related prosthetic joint infections. Adv Exp Med Biol 2017;973:31–9.

70. Drago L, Signori V, De Vecchi E, et al. Use of dithiothreitol to improve the diagnosis of prosthetic joint infections. J Orthop Res 2013;31:1694–9.

71. Romano CL, Trentinaglia MT, De Vecchi E, et al. Cost-benefit analysis of antibiofilm microbiological techniques for peri-prosthetic joint infection diagnosis. BMC Infect Dis 2018;18:1–10.

72. Veeh RH, Shirtliff ME, Petik JR, et al. Detection of *Staphylococcus aureus* biofilm on tampons and menses components. J Infect Dis 2003;188:519–30.

73. Nistico L, Gieseke A, Stoodley P, et al. Fluorescence "in situ" hybridization for the detection of biofilm in the middle ear and upper respiratory tract mucosa. Methods Mol Biol 2009;493:191–213.

74. Costerton JW, Post JC, Ehrlich GD, et al. New methods for the detection of orthopedic and other biofilm infections. FEMS Immunol Med Microbiol 2011;61:133–40.

75. Ecker DJ, Sampath R, Massire C, et al. Ibis T5000: a universal biosensor approach for microbiology. Nat Rev Microbiol 2008;6:553–8.

76. Palmer MP, Melton-Kreft R, Nistico L, et al. Polymerase chain reaction-electrospray-time of flight mass spectrometry versus culture for bacterial detection in septic arthritis and osteoarthritis. Genet Test Mol Biomarkers 2016;20:721–31.

77. Available at: FDA.gov. Accessed July 22, 2018.

78. BioFire Diagnostics. Available at: http://www.bio-firedx.com. Accessed July 22, 2018.

79. Khare R, Espy MJ, Cebelinski E, et al. Comparative evaluation of two commercial multiplex panels for detection of gastrointestinal pathogens by use of clinical stool specimens. J Clin Microbiol 2014;52:3667–73.

80. Bode LGM, Kluytmans JAJW, Wertheim HFL, et al. Preventing surgical-site infection in nasal carriers of *Staphylococcus aureus*. N Engl J Med 2010;362:9–17.

81. Wyatt MC, Beswick AD, Kunutsor ST, et al. The alpha-defensin immunoassay and leukocyte esterase colorimetric strip test for the diagnosis of periprosthetic joint infection: a systematic review and meta-analysis. J Bone Joint Surg Am 2016;98:992–1000.

82. De Vecchi E, Villa F, Bortolin M, et al. Leucocyte esterase, glucose and C-reactive protein in the diagnosis of prosthetic joint infections: a prospective study. Clin Microbiol Infect 2016;22:555–60.

83. Alvand A, Rezapoor M, Parvizi J. The role of biomarkers for the diagnosis of implant-related infections in orthopaedics and trauma. Adv Exp Med Biol 2017;971:69–79.

84. Deirmengian C, Kardos K, Kilmartin P, et al. Diagnosing periprosthetic joint infection: has the era of the biomarker arrived? Clin Orthop Relat Res 2014;472:3254–62.

85. Stone WZ, Gray CF, Parvataneni HK, et al. Clinical evaluation of synovial alpha defensing and synovial C-reactive protein in the diagnosis of periprosthetic joint infection. J Bone Joint Surg Am 2018;100:1184–9.

86. Brinker MR, O'Connor DP. Nonunions: evaluation and treatment. In: Browner BD, Jupiter JB, Krettek C, et al, editors. Skeletal trauma. 5th edition. Philadelphia: Elsevier Saunders; 2015. p. 637–718.

Pediatrics

New Technologies in Pediatric Spine Surgery

Yasser Ibrahim Alkhalife, MBBS, SB (Orth),
Kedar Prashant Padhye, MBBS, DNB (Ortho), Ron El-Hawary, MD, MSc, FRCS(C)*

KEYWORDS

- AIS • EOS • Fusionless • Thoracoscopic • MCGR • Posterior dynamic deformity correction
- Apifix • Trolley

KEY POINTS

- Spinal fusion in young children for treatment of early-onset scoliosis is not optimal because it limits growth and contributes to long-term lung compromise.
- Fusion decreases spinal mobility and may lead to development of adjacent level disc degeneration in healthy teenagers for the treatment of adolescent idiopathic scoliosis.
- Magnetically controlled growing rod and the modern Luque trolley are newer, growth-friendly methods to minimize the number of surgeries and hopefully the number of complications in the management of early-onset scoliosis.
- A variety of different new technologies that halt curve progression, while maintaining spinal mobility have been studied, including vertebral body tethering and posterior dynamic deformity correction.

INTRODUCTION

Early-onset scoliosis (EOS) is a spine deformity that is present before 10 years of age.[1] EOS has many potential etiologies (congenital or structural, neuromuscular, syndromic, and idiopathic). A novel classification system for EOS has been developed and consists of continuous age prefix, etiology, major curve angle, kyphosis, and an optional progression modifier.[2] Because the treatment principles for children between the ages of 5 and 10 years more closely resemble those used for children under the age of 5 years, 10 years of age has been agreed on to be a logical age to differentiate between EOS and late-onset scoliosis.[3]

Spinal fusion in young children for treatment of EOS is not optimal because it limits thoracic growth and contributes to long-term lung compromise. Various types of growth-friendly spinal implants have been introduced and these systems fall into 3 categories based on the forces of correction they exert on the spine. Distraction-based systems correct spinal deformities by mechanically applying a distractive force across a deformed segment with anchors at the proximal and distal of the implants, which commonly attach to the spine, rib, and/or pelvis. Examples of traditional distraction-based implants are spine-based or rib-based growing rods, including traditional growing rods, vertical expandable titanium rib prosthesis, and, more recently, magnetically controlled growing rods. Compression-based systems correct spinal deformities with a compressive force applied to the convexity of the curve, causing growth inhibition of the convex side. Examples of compression-based systems are vertebral body staples and vertebral body tethering. Guided growth systems correct spinal deformity by

---

This research did not receive any specific grant from funding agencies in the public, commercial, or not-for-profit sectors.

Division of Orthopaedic Surgery, IWK Health Centre, PO Box 9700, 5850 University Avenue, Halifax, Nova Scotia, B3K-6R8 Canada

* Corresponding author.

E-mail address: ron.el-hawary@iwk.nshealth.ca

anchoring multiple and apical vertebrae to rods with mechanical forces including translation at the time of the initial implantation. The majority of the anchors are not rigidly attached to the rods, thus permitting longitudinal growth over time as the anchors slide over the rods. An example of guided growth systems is the Shilla system (Medtronic, Memphis, TN).[4]

High complication rates are associated with fusionless growing rod treatment in patients with EOS. The management of EOS is prolonged; therefore, complications are frequent and should be expected. Complications include wound complications, prominent implants, alignment issues, and unplanned surgical procedures.[5] Magnetically controlled growing rods and the modern Luque trolley (MLT) are newer methods to intended to minimize the number of surgeries and hopefully the number of complications in the management of EOS.[6–10]

Adolescent idiopathic scoliosis (AIS) is a structural lateral curvature of the spine with a significant rotatory component that starts to be clinically apparent in healthy teenagers around the pubertal growth spurt. Some feel that individuals with curves up to 20° to 25° can be managed with scoliosis-specific exercises, such as the Schroth method, whereas curves between 25° and 40° are often braced with a thoracolumbar spinal orthosis.[9] The BrAIST study showed the effectiveness of bracing in preventing curves from reaching 50° at skeletal maturity in the majority of patients.[11] However, bracing is not always successful at controlling scoliosis and sometimes psychosocial and practical issues may limit the success of bracing in some individuals.[11,12] Failure of bracing with curves reaching 50°, especially in young patients, may ultimately continue to progress and result in traditional surgical intervention with a spinal fusion. Fusion remains a viable option, but decreases spinal mobility and may lead to the development of adjacent level disc degeneration.[13,14] Thus, there remains a practical need to develop motion-sparing, fusionless technologies. Because of the issues with bracing and with spinal fusion, surgeons have searched for alternative approaches that halt curve progression while maintaining spinal mobility.[15–18] A variety of different new technologies have been studied, including vertebral body tethering and posterior dynamic deformity correction.[9,10]

The aim of this article is to elaborate in detail the indications, contraindications, operative techniques, early outcomes, and complications associated with these new technologies.

NORMAL SPINAL GROWTH
General Principles

Growth is a major factor that should be taken into account with scoliosis.[19] Knowledge of normal growth parameters allows a better understanding of abnormal spine growth and of the pathologic changes induced in the growing spine by an early-onset spinal deformity.[20]

During growth, complex phenomena follow each other in very rapid succession. These events are well-synchronized to maintain harmonious limb and spine relationships because growth does not occur simultaneously in the same magnitude or rate in the various body segments.[20] The slightest error or modification can lead to a malformation or deformity with negative effects on standing and sitting height, thoracic cage shape, volume and circumference, and lung development.[19–23] All types of growth are interrelated. Thus, as the spinal deformity progresses by a "domino effect," not only is spinal growth affected, but also the size and shape of the thoracic cage are modified. Over time, the scoliotic disorder changes in nature and from a mainly orthopedic issue, it becomes a severe pediatric, systemic disorder with thoracic insufficiency syndrome,[24,25] cor pulmonale,[26] and reduced body mass index. In most severe cases, these alterations can be lethal.[19–23]

Height and Weight Measurements

A thorough analysis of standing and sitting height, arm span, weight, thoracic perimeter, T1 to S1 spinal segment length, and respiratory function help the surgeon to plan the best treatment at the right time.[27] Standing height is a global marker and consists of 2 specific measurements, the subischial height (leg length) and the sitting height. The gain in standing height is approximately 25 cm during the first year of life and around 12.5 cm during the second year. Between ages 2 and 3 and 3 and 4 years, the gain in standing height is approximately 9 cm/y and 7 cm/y, respectively. At 5 years of age, standing height increases by 5.0 to 5.5 cm each year in both boys and girls. At the onset of puberty, the remaining growth is about 18 cm for girls and 20 cm for boys.[20]

The sitting height averages 34 cm at birth and averages 88 cm for girls for a standing height of 1.65 cm and 92.00 cm for boys at the end of growth for a standing height of 1.75 m.[19] In children with severe spinal deformities, loss of sitting height is related to the severity of the deformity. For this reason, it is important to monitor changes in the sitting height rather than in the standing height in children with scoliosis. The measurement of sitting height can also be useful in anticipating the onset of puberty. When the sitting height is approximately 84 cm, 80% of girls have menarche.[28]

Weight is a useful parameter for analyzing growth and increases by 20-fold from birth to skeletal maturity. At 5 years of age, weight is approximately 20 kg, 30 kg by 10 years, and reaches 60 kg or more by 16 years. It should be kept in mind also that the during pubertal spurt, weight usually doubles.[28]

Many spinal deformities originate in T1 to S1 spinal segment. It should be recalled that the height of the spine accounts for 60% of total sitting height, with the head and the pelvis accounting for the remaining 40%.[28] The T1 to S1 segment accounts for approximately 50% of the sitting height, two-thirds for the thoracic spine and one-third for the lumbar spine.[20]

The thoracic spine makes up 30% of the sitting height, and a single thoracic vertebra and its disc represent about 2.5% of sitting height.[20] A precocious arthrodesis of this segment has effects on thoracic growth and lung development.[29,30] The lumbar spine makes up about 18% of the sitting height, and a single lumbar vertebra and its disc represent 3.5% of sitting height.[28]

Thoracic Growth

Thoracic volume has been called the fourth dimension of the spine. At birth, the thoracic cage volume is approximately 6% of its final size and reaches 30% by age 5 and 50% by age 10. Between age 10 and skeletal maturity, the thoracic cage volume doubles before it ultimately stops growing. The "golden" period for both thoracic spine and thoracic cage growth occurs between birth and 8 years of age and coincides with lung development. It is important to preserve both thoracic growth and lung volume during this critical period of life.[28]

Gollogly and colleagues[31] showed that lung parenchyma volume is a function of age. There were 1050 normal computed tomography scans of the chest with 3-dimensional volumetric reconstruction of the pulmonary system that were reviewed and, at birth, the lung parenchyma volume is 400 mL, approximately 900 and 1500 mL at ages 5 and 10 years, respectively, and around 4500 mL for boys and 3500 mL for girls at skeletal maturity.

Phases of Growth Spurt

Puberty starts at 13 years for boys (bone age). The ascending side (acceleration phase) lasts from 13 to 15 years of bone age. This period corresponds with peak growth and it is not a single point. It lasts for 2 years and, during this period, the gain in standing height is 16.5 cm. The gain in sitting height is ±8.5 cm. The gain in subischial length is 8 cm. The triradiate cartilage closes 1 year after the onset of puberty and the ascending phase is approximately 14 years of bone age.[32–42]

The descending side (deceleration phase) is characterized by a steady decrease in velocity of annual growth. It lasts 3 years from 15 to 18 years of age. The remaining growth in standing height is approximately 6 cm: 4.1 cm in sitting height and 1.9 cm in subischial length. During this phase, the trunk grows more than the lower limb, which stops growing at Risser 1.

Puberty starts at 11 years of bone age for girls. At the beginning of puberty, the average remaining growth in standing height is approximately 20.5 cm. The gain in the sitting height is approximately 11.5 cm. The gain in subischial length is approximately 9 cm. The ascending phase (acceleration phase) starts from 11 to 13 years of bone age. The peak growth lasts for 2 years and during this phase, the gain in standing height is 15.1 cm (±1 cm); in sitting height it is 7.7 cm (±0.5 cm), and in subischial height it is 7.4 cm (±0.5 cm). The triradiate cartilage closes 1 year after the beginning of puberty, at approximately 12 years of bone age.[32–42]

The descending phase (deceleration phase) is characterized by a steady decrease in the annual velocity of growth. It lasts for 3 years, from 13 to 16 years of age. The remaining growth is approximately 5.4 cm in standing height with 3.8 cm in sitting height and 1.6 cm in subischial length. The lower limb stops going after menarche. This equals our Risser 1. Menarche occurs on the descending side of puberty: 42% of the girl's experience menarche before Risser 1, 31% at Risser 1, 13% at Risser 2, 8% at Risser 3, and 5% at Risser 4. After 2 years of menarche, there is usually no more growth.[32–42]

NEW TECHNOLOGIES IN PEDIATRIC SPINE SURGERY

Various types of growth-friendly spinal implants and newer technologies have been introduced in the past few years to avoid long-term lung compromise in young children with EOS treated with spinal fusion. Similarly, in AIS, a variety of different new technologies have been developed that halt curve progression, while maintaining spinal mobility to minimize adjacent level disc degeneration that can result from spinal fusion.

Magnetically Controlled Growing Rods

The initial proof of concept for a remote-controlled growing spinal rod for the correction of scoliosis was in 5 beagle dogs in 1998.[43] The MAGEC system (NuVasive, San Diego, CA) is a type of magnetically controlled growing rods and is a novel technology used in the surgical management of EOS. This system approved by the US Food and Drug Administration (FDA). It is a distraction-based spinal implants, which can lengthen without surgery and may theoretically have the benefit of minimizing many complications resulting from surgery, such as infection and soft tissue problems. Because the device can be adjusted magnetically, lengthening can be performed in most cases in an outpatient setting without anesthesia or sedation.

Implant design

The MAGEC system consists of 1 or 2 sterile and single-use titanium implantable growth rods and an external remote control for noninvasive lengthening. The diameter of the rods used varies depending on the child's body weight (4.5 mm for children weighing up to 27 kg, 5.5 mm for children weighing up to 36 kg). A 6-mm rod is also available as an alternative option. A portion of each MAGEC rod contains a telescopic distraction element, the actuator, which includes an internal cylindrical rare earth magnet. There are 70-mm and 90-mm actuators that have potential lengthening of 28 mm and 48 mm, respectively. The system also includes a manual distractor (to check the implant is functional before implantation) and a wand locator (to locate the internal magnet).

Authors' preferred procedure technique

Under general anesthesia, all patients are carefully positioned prone on top of a radiolucent table. All bony prominences are well-padded and the posterior spine is prepared and draped. All surgeries should be performed using comprehensive intraoperative neuromonitoring. Under fluoroscopic guidance, the most proximal and distal vertebral levels of instrumentation are marked and 2 separate longitudinal incisions are performed at these levels. After dissection, laminar hooks and/or pedicle screws are inserted proximally and screws distally to create upper and lower fused foundations. Before insertion, each rod is tested intraoperatively with a sterile magnet to make sure that the magnetic driver is functioning. The rod can be contoured in the sagittal plane except for the actuator portion, which cannot be contoured

and should be placed at thoracolumbar junction. The rods have the options of standard-standard or standard-offset orientation. In a fashion similar to traditional growing rods, the rods are inserted in the submuscular layer and connected to the anchors provided. The instrumented levels are decorticated between the screws or hooks to encourage local fusion at the anchor points. Once the rods are placed and secured, final confirmatory anterior–posterior and lateral fluoroscopic views are taken and a thorough irrigation with saline is performed. The wounds are closed in a standard manner (Figs. 1–3).

Postoperative protocol

At our institution, patients are evaluated every 3 months to perform outpatient distraction. The frequency of distraction is the topic of study of an upcoming multicenter, randomized, controlled trial that is a combined effort between the Children's Spine Study Group and the Growing Spine Study Group. Patients will be randomized to distractions at either 6-week or 16-week intervals. Regardless of the frequency, distraction is performed with the patient positioned prone on an examining table through the external remote control placed externally over the patient's spine at the location of the actuator portion of the rod. The rods are identified with a small magnet and the rods are lengthened simultaneously. The rods can be lengthened to maximal allowable by the stiffness of the tissues (ie, until kickback or "clunk" is felt) or to a predetermined length as estimated by normalized age-matched growth. The distractions are performed in an outpatient setting without the need for anesthesia or sedation. Verification of the new rod length is performed using either ultrasound examination or radiography (Figs. 4 and 5).

Review of the literature

Numerous early studies have reported the short-term effectiveness of the magnetically controlled growing rods. Cheung and colleagues[44] were the first authors to describe early clinical results of the magnetically controlled growing rod technique that did not require open lengthening like traditional growing rods.

Akbarnia and colleagues[6] reported preliminary findings from a prospective, observational, multicenter study involving 14 children with EOS who received magnetically controlled growing rods. The mean preoperative Cobb angle was 60°. Postoperatively, the mean Cobb angle was 34° initially and 31° at the latest follow-up. The mean number of distractions

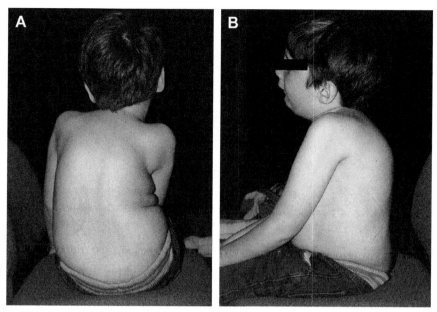

Fig. 1. (A, B) Clinical pictures of an 8-year-old boy with spinal muscle atrophy type II and early-onset scoliosis. Note the scoliosis, upper thoracic kyphosis, pelvic obliquity, and chest wall deformities.

per child was 4.9 and the mean preoperative total spine height increased from 292 mm preoperatively to 322 mm postoperatively and 338 mm at final follow-up. No significant differences in the Cobb angle correction were found between children receiving single or dual rods.

Dannawi and colleagues[45] reported a prospective case series involving 34 children receiving magnetically controlled growing rods. The mean preoperative Cobb angle was 69°. This angle decreased to a mean of 47° postoperatively and to 41° at final reported follow-up. The mean preoperative total spine height was

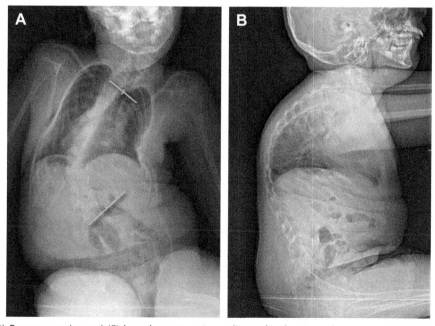

Fig. 2. (A) Posteroanterior and (B) lateral preoperative radiographs showing a long sweeping curve and pelvic obliquity of neuromuscular early-onset scoliosis.

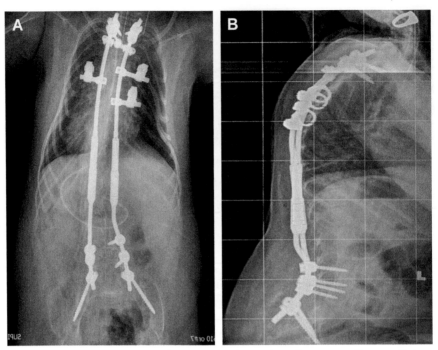

Fig. 3. Postoperative (*A*) posteroanterior and (*B*) lateral radiographs with magnetically controlled growing rods inserted.

304 mm: this increased to 335 mm immediately after surgery and to 348 mm at final review. The mean number of distractions per child was 4.8.

La Rosa and colleagues[46] reported preliminary findings from a study involving 10 children receiving magnetically controlled growing rods. The average curve correction was 57.7% of the initial scoliosis angle. Two patients experienced rod breakage and 1 patient had a pull-out of 2 hooks at the top of the construct 9 months after surgery. No intraoperative complications occurred and no surgical site infections or other complications were recorded. The authors stated that, although implant-related complications could occur, as in all EOS growing rods procedures, magnetically controlled growing rods can be used effectively in patients with EOS and can overcome surgical scarring, surgical site infection, and psychological distress owing to multiple surgeries needed in the traditional growing rods system (Table 1).

Modern Luque Trolley

The MLT is a recently developed growth guidance system to provide spinal deformity correction and to allow for growth of the children's immature spine without requiring repetitive lengthening interventions. The MLT solution is based on the concept introduced by Luque[47] to guide spinal growth along a given trajectory. However, it allows for the application of a growth-guiding construct without the use of sublaminar or cerclage wires. The MLT consists of gliding spinal anchors traveling along fixed, overlapping rods, preventing further spinal deformity while still allowing relatively normal spinal growth. These anchors are inserted through muscle-sparing extraperiosteal "keyhole" dissections to avoid spontaneous fusion. The anchors are placed for maximal apical translation and deformity correction at the apex of the deformity.[7]

The highly polished titanium rods are designed for gliding in combination with TROLLEY gliding vehicles. The cable tie is made from polyetheretherketone and provides a low profile. The bearing surfaces of the MLT are made from ultra-high molecular weight polyethylene, reducing material wear while allowing for gliding of the rods (Fig. 6).

Authors' preferred procedure technique

After induction of general anesthesia, the patient is placed in a prone position on the flat top of a radiolucent table with all bony prominences well-padded. A single midline incision spanning the segment of the spine to be instrumented is made with multiple keyhole transmuscular dissections for the gliding anchors and a

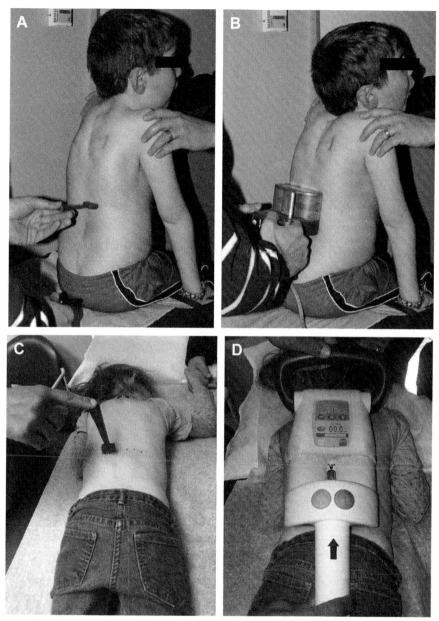

Fig. 4. (A, B) Subsequent distractions are performed in an outpatient setting without the need for anesthesia or sedation. (C, D) Another example of subsequent distractions being performed prone in a different patient. ([D] *Courtesy of* NuVasive, San Diego, CA.)

subperiosteal dissection for distal and/or proximal anchor fusions. The surgical technique consists of gliding spinal anchors taking advantage of muscle-sparing, minimally invasive exposure to avoid spontaneous fusion. Fluoroscopic guidance confirms the pedicle entry point and, using a freehand technique, the gliding screws are inserted at strategic points allowing maximal apical translation. Two pairs of 5- or 6-mm titanium rods are tunneled in a subfascial/ intramuscular fashion (below the fascia, above the periosteum) from the opened proximal and distal ends. Each rod had only 1 end rigidly anchored to the spine. In the intermediate segments, a series of gliding spinal anchors maintain the correction by keeping the rods parallel and engaged. As the spine grows, the rigidly proximal-fixed rods move away from the distally fixed rods. The number of gliding anchorage points was kept to a minimum to minimize the

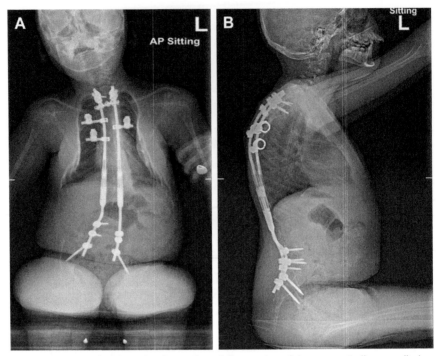

Fig. 5. (A) Posteroanterior and (B) lateral radiographs at full excursion of the magnetically controlled growing rods pending exchange.

risk of spontaneous fusion, yet an adequate number of gliding anchors was necessary to translate the apex of the deformity toward the midline to control and correct the spinal deformity. Postoperatively, patients were mobilized on days 1 to 2. No specific physiotherapy was initiated and return to regular activities was recommended by 6 months after surgery. All patients were seen at a regular postoperative visit at 6 weeks, 12 weeks, and then at 6-month intervals until they reached skeletal maturity (Figs. 7–9).

Review of the literature
Ouellet and colleagues[48] recently presented their first experimental animal study results about MLT construct in an immature animal model. These studies to determine biological compatibility, stability, and growth potential of the trolley gliding vehicle were used in a novel surgical technique for guided spinal growth. The gliding spinal anchors evaluated in this study demonstrated a high potential for self-lengthening as a treatment option for EOS. Implant loosening was likely mechanical because no signs of reactive inflammatory reaction were found. Reducing heterotrophic ossification and spontaneous facet arthrodesis remains a challenge in managing the immature spine. The trolley gliding vehicle is not FDA approved and questions remain about the effect of wear debris and the risk of spontaneous fusions.[7]

Table 1	
Authors' preferred indications and contraindications for using magnetically controlled growing rods	
Authors' Preferred Indications	**Authors' Preferred Contraindications**
1. Progressive early-onset scoliosis with failed nonoperative treatment (P2 annual progression ratio of 10° progression over 6 mo (P2 is annual progression ratio of >20°/year))[2] 2. Cobb angle of >45°	1. Skeletally mature 2. Patients with infections or pathologic conditions of bone that would impair the ability to securely fix the device 3. Patients with a pacemaker or other active, electronic devices 4. Patients <2 y old 5. Body weight of <25 lb (11.4 kg) 6. Patients with stainless steel wires or other implants containing incompatible material

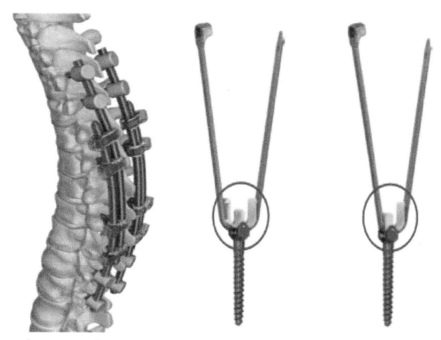

Fig. 6. The modern Luque trolley system with the bearing surfaces made from ultra-high molecular weight polyethylene, reducing material wear while allowing for gliding of the rods. (*CGI Artwork courtesy of* pixelmolkerei.ch.)

Ouellet in 2011[7] published a small series of 17 patients with EOS, of whom 5 were treated with an early version of the MLT construct. The mean preoperative Cobb angle of the primary curve was corrected from 60° (range, 45°–70°) to 21° (range, 15°–32°). Over the course of 4.5 years, the mean Cobb angle had gradually increased to 31° (range, 14°–54°); 2 patients outgrew their

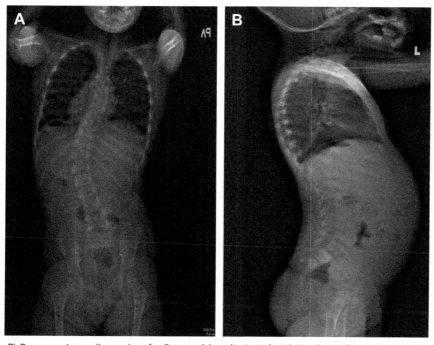

Fig. 7. (*A*, *B*) Preoperative radiographs of a 5-year-old scoliotic girl with Prader–Willi syndrome with early-onset scoliosis.

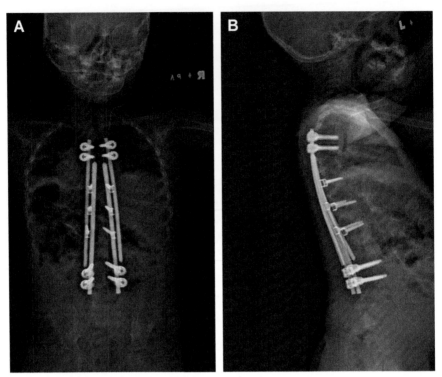

Fig. 8. Immediate postoperative (A) posteroanterior and (B) lateral radiographs with the modern Luque trolley.

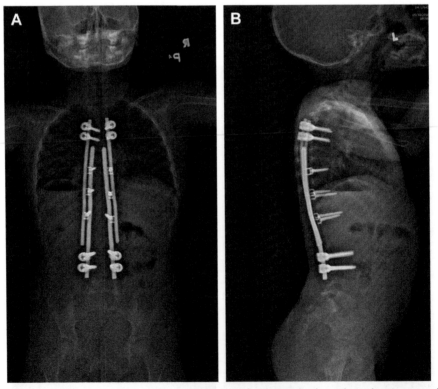

Fig. 9. Postoperative (1 year) (A) posteroanterior and (B) lateral radiographs the with modern Luque trolley. Note the growth achieved by the distance between the free tips of each of the 4 rods from the end vertebral pedicle screw foundations has increased as compared with immediately postoperatively.

initial constructs and required revision surgery. One patient had a Cobb angle regression close to its initial value and demonstrated little spinal growth. All 3 underwent revision surgery. The remaining 2 patients continued to grow with no evidence of curve regression. Intraoperative findings demonstrated persistent gliding motion across the 3 gliding screws and at the sublaminar cables. In keeping with motion, particle debris was noted at the rod–screw interface as well as at the cable–rod interface. All 5 patients' postoperative courses were uneventful and there were no superficial or deep wound infections or rod breakage. However, radiographs did reveal that 3 sublaminar cables ruptured in 2 patients, but without any clinical consequences. This concept is quite new and, therefore, further long-term results of the clinical studies are needed (Table 2).

Vertebral Body Tethering

Vertebral body tethering was first described in a 2010 case report published by Crawford and Lenke.[18] This novel method for spinal growth modulation with a flexible spinal implant has the potential to avoid progression of the deformity during the adolescent growth spurt. The concept is to stop the vertebral growth on the convexity of the scoliosis. This dynamic epiphysiodesis of the convexity aims to equilibrate the height of both concave and convex sides of the vertebra without fusion.[49] The biomechanical basis for growth modulation via a flexible tether has been demonstrated in animal models. Newton and colleagues[16,17] demonstrated that, in an immature porcine model, a flexible polyethylene tether attached via pedicle screws along the anterolateral aspect of the spine could alter spinal morphology and induce a scoliotic deformity. Braun and colleagues[50] have demonstrated similar results in a goat model. At this time of publication, specific medical devices developed for this technique are not FDA approved for skeletally immature patients.

Authors' preferred procedure technique

Surgery is performed under general anesthesia with a double-lumen tube and single-lung ventilation. By deflating the lung on the convex side of the scoliosis, better visibility of the spine is achieved, which should allow for a safer and more technically easier surgery. After intubation, an arterial line, urinary catheter, and electrodes for intraoperative neuromonitoring are inserted. The patient is positioned in a lateral decubitus position on a radiolucent table with the convex side up. All bony prominences are well-padded and an axillary gel role is placed under the patient. The whole procedure is performed with video-assisted thoracoscopy. The vertebrae of the main curve are identified with C-arm fluoroscopy in the anteroposterior and the lateral projections. We prefer 2 mid-axillary anterior portals (12 mm) and 3 posterior working portals (15 mm) through the intercostal spaces. First, a superoanterior portal is used to visualize the chest cavity. At this point, the lung is deflated to better visualize the vertebral column. A 30° scope is inserted in the superoanterior portal to visualize the extent of the exposure. The parietal pleura is dissected off the lateral aspect of the vertebral bodies at all levels in sequential fashion from the upper end to the lower end vertebrae along the length of the curve (Fig. 10A). Once the pleura has been incised for the length of spine to be tethered, the segmental vessels are identified and coagulated with a harmonic blade (Fig. 10B). We prefer to wait at least 15 to 20 minutes per level of segmental sacrificed to ensure that there are not any changes in the intraoperative neurophysiologic monitoring.

Care is taken to ensure that the disk spaces remain untouched to avoid unwanted fusion. Rib heads can be prominent at T5 to T7 and sometimes need resection before insertion of staples and screws. A 3-prong staple is placed in the anterior aspect of the vertebral body

Table 2 Authors' preferred indications and contraindications for using the Modern Luque Trolley	
Authors' Preferred Indications	Authors' Preferred Contraindications
1. Spinal deformity (Cobb >40°–50°) 2. Failed nonoperative treatment (curve progression >10° over a 6-mo interval) 3. Considerable growth potential defined by prepeak growth velocity, bone age <10; open triradiate cartilage 4. Age 5–10 y with an expected significant spinal deformity of >80° at skeletal maturity	1. Patients with chest wall abnormalities contributing to thoracic insufficiency syndrome 2. Rigid kyphoscoliosis 3. Cobb >100° or bends <50° 4. Skeletally mature 5. Prior spinal surgery

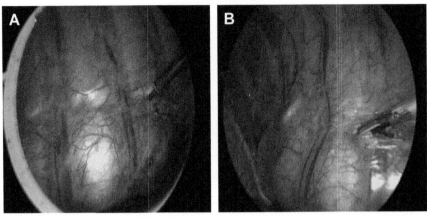

Fig. 10. (A) The parietal pleura is dissected off the lateral aspect of the vertebral bodies. (B) The segmental vessels are identified and coagulated with a harmonic blade.

adjacent to the rib head. Sequentially at all levels, screws of appropriate size are inserted (Fig. 11). As we insert the awl/staple, tap, and screw, we are verifying anterior to posterior position with the "pipeline" view of the thoracoscope. Simultaneously, we are verifying superior to inferior position with anteroposterior fluoroscopy. Care is taken to remain just anterior to the rib head to ensure that the staple is not in the foramen. Subsequently, the screw hole is tapped under fluoroscopic guidance aiming for the contralateral rib head and then the screw is placed. Proper position is again checked and confirmed using portable fluoroscopy. At each level, once the screw is inserted a tether is placed in the tulip of each screw sequentially and set screw is used to secure the tether (Fig. 12). We prefer to tension the tether at each level sequentially as we insert screws.

Correction of the curve occurs through both tensioning of the tether and translation of the spine. Residual tether is trimmed leaving at least 2 cm at both ends to accommodate potential future lengthening (Fig. 13).

At the end of the procedure, a thorough irrigation of the hemithorax with saline is performed and an appropriate size chest tube is inserted into the lowest of the posterior portals through a subcutaneous tunnel, 1 interspace cranial to the incision. The lung is then reinflated under direct vision and the incisions are closed in layers with the chest tube connected to 20 cm H_2O of suction.

Postoperative protocol
The chest tube is removed at day 2. Chest physiotherapy with incentive spirometry is encouraged. A chest radiograph is taken daily for the

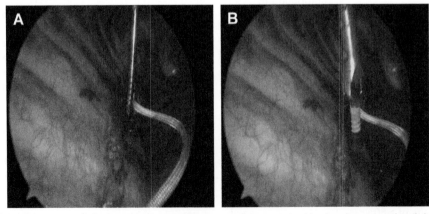

Fig. 11. (A) A 3-prong staple is placed in the anterior aspect of the vertebral body adjacent to the rib head before tapping the vertebral body. (B) The screw is placed.

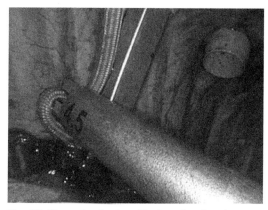

Fig. 12. The tether is placed in the tulip of each screw sequentially and a set screw is used to secure the tether.

first 3 postoperative days to rule out atelectasis, pneumothorax, or hemothorax. Activities as tolerated are gradually introduced once the chest tube is removed.

Review of the literature

Crawford and Lenke[18] reported on a skeletally immature patient who underwent anterior vertebral body tethering and demonstrated progressive correction of his curvature over a 5-year time span. Anterior vertebral body tethering has been extensively studied in animal models. Newton and colleagues[16,17] have demonstrated the ability of a unilateral tether to induce deformity in a bovine model with radiographic evidence of disc wedging and rotation, while retaining spine flexibility. Braun and colleagues[50] have demonstrated similar results in a goat model.

Samdani and colleagues[51] reported on their first 32 consecutive patients treated with

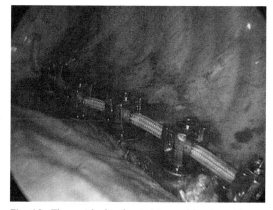

Fig. 13. The residual tether is trimmed leaving at least 2 cm at both ends to accommodate potential future lengthening.

anterior vertebral body tethering in the thoracic spine. The mean age was 12 years and patients were skeletally immature, with a mean Risser score of 0.42. The mean operating room time was 286.2 minutes. The preoperative main thoracic Cobb angle averaged 42.8° ± 8.0°, with a compensatory lumbar curve of 25.2° ± 7.3° and a proximal thoracic curve of 22.8° ± 7.9°. On first erect radiograph, these corrected to main thoracic 21.0° ± 8.5°, lumbar 18.0° ± 7.1°, and proximal thoracic 14.4° ± 7.6°. At last follow-up, the main thoracic and lumbar curves improved to 17.9° ± 11.4° and 12.6° ± 9.4°, respectively. Sagittal plane parameters remained stable. Overall, the patients' thoracic scoliometer readings improved from a preoperative value of 13.4° to most recent value of 7.4°. Preoperatively, 88% of patients had a rib prominence measuring greater than 10°. At most recent follow-up, only 28% of patients had a measurement greater than 10°. No neurologic, infectious, or hardware-related complications occurred. One patient had persistent atelectasis that required a bronchoscopy.

A 2-year follow-up of this technique was reported in 11 skeletally immature patients with idiopathic scoliosis. The mean age was 12.3 ± 1.6 years and the preoperative thoracic Cobb angle averaged 44.2° ± 9.0° and corrected to 20.3° ± 11.0° on first erect, with progressive improvement at 2 years to 13.5° ± 11.6°. Similarly, the preoperative lumbar curve of 25.1° + 8.7° demonstrated progressive correction on first erect to 14.9° ± 4.9° and to 7.2° ± 5.1° at 2 years. No major complications were observed and 2 patients returned to the operating room at 2 years postoperatively for loosening of the tether to prevent overcorrection.[10]

Boudissa and colleagues[52] reported on 6 patients with a mean age of 11.2 ± 1.2 years (range, 9–12 years). The mean follow-up was 21.6 months (range, 18–24 months), the mean main thoracic curvature before surgery was 45° ± 10° (range, 35°–60°), and the mean lumbar curvature was 33° ± 5° (range, 30°–40°). Correction of the main thoracic curvature and the mean lumbar curvature was 38° ± 7° (range, 30°–50°) and 23° ± 6° (range, 15°–30°), respectively. They reported that all patients were well-balanced in the frontal plan and the sagittal plane on full spine radiographs and no complications or overcorrection were recorded (Table 3).

Posterior Dynamic Deformity Correction

Postoperative spinal motion is significantly diminished owing to the fusion of the spine with standard surgical techniques.[53] In addition,

Table 3
Authors' preferred indications and contraindications for using vertebral body tethering

Authors' Preferred Indications	Authors' Preferred Contraindications
1. Cobb angle 40–65°	1. Age <10 y
2. Flexibility below 35°	2. Risser ≥3
3. Single thoracic curve	3. >40° of thoracic kyphosis
4. Single lumbar curve	4. Rib prominences >20°
5. Double major curves	
6. Age >10 y	
7. Risser 0–2	
8. Kyphosis <40°	

patients who undergo fusion surgery report a lower physical function as compared with non-scoliotic controls at long-term follow-up, which could be attributed to the invasive surgery and stiffening of the spine.[54] A new, less invasive device with fewer instrumented segments is the posterior dynamic deformity correction device (ApiFix Ltd, Misgav, Israel).[9] The unique features of the device allow spinal instrumentation without fusion.

Implant design

The device has an overall length range of 85 to 125 mm, and is expanded in increments of 1.3 mm, for total extension of 30 to 40 mm, depending on length (Fig. 14). The device has a miniratchet mechanism that allows unidirectional elongation of an expandable rod. The miniratchet mechanism consists of a toothed area and a locking tooth, which are both made from a titanium alloy. The locking tooth rotates around a 2-mm pin and interacts with the toothed area to allow only unidirectional movement. The locking tooth is pressed via a flat spring to prevent slippage. The spring portion is made from nitinol. The remainder of the device is made from titanium alloy with an amorphous diamond-like ceramic coating, which is designed to minimize friction and wear. The ceramic coating also has the potential to inhibit bacterial growth, which may decrease the incidence of postoperative deep wound infections. The expandable rod with polyaxial rings at its extremities is attached by 2 pedicle screws around the apex of the main spinal curvature. Rod expansion is incremental and gradual, making the deformity correction safer than "all at once" acute rod distraction in the standard-type surgery. Spanning the correction process over several weeks or months allows the soft tissues to accommodate any incremental correction. The long, incremental process decreases the load on the screws and allows the body to slowly rebuild itself in the correct position/shape.

The implant also has a control pin that can abort the ratchet mechanism and put the device in a free neutral mode or a locked position, creating a stiff fusion-like rod. The device is a

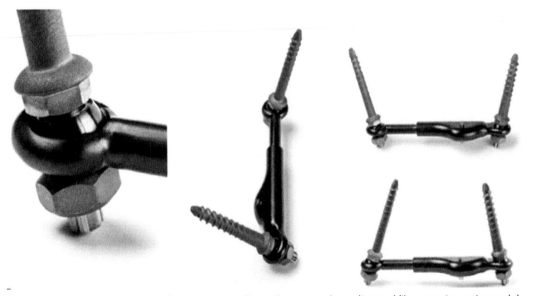

Fig. 14. The ApiFix system is made from a titanium alloy with an amorphous diamond-like ceramic coating and the spring part is made from nitinol. (*Courtesy of* ApiFix, Ltd, Misgav, Israel.)

unilateral construct that connects 2 periapical pedicle screws through polyaxial mobile ball-and-socket joints with a rod. The device is inserted on the concave side of the curve. The rod includes a ratchet that can elongate when the patient performs exercises after surgery, especially with side bending toward the convexity. By side bending, the ratchet allows elongation of the rod and thereby corrects the scoliotic curve. The ratchet does not allow for shortening when the patient stands upright again and, thus, it preserves the correction. The polyaxial joints allow the pedicle screws to have a range of motion of 30° (15° per pedicle screw) in flexion, extension, and axial rotation.

Authors' preferred procedure technique
After induction of general anesthesia and endotracheal intubation, the patient is positioned prone on the spine top of the radiolucent table. All bony prominences are well-padded. Intraoperative neuromonitoring should be used. Halo femoral traction is preferred because it aids with correction. The posterior spine is prepared and draped in the usual manner. Under the guidance of portable fluoroscopy, the landmarks of the pedicles on the concave side of the curve are identified. The contralateral side is left undisturbed. A midline skin incision is used (in case of a large curve, 2 small skin incisions can be used, exposing the end vertebrae using a minimally invasive surgical technique). Subcutaneous tissue is dissected in line with the skin incision. The fascia is then incised in the midline and subperiosteal dissection is performed to expose the tips of the transverse processes of the desired vertebrae. Pedicle screws are inserted at the desired vertebral levels. In cases of longer curves, device extenders can be used on either end of the device. The device is then connected to the pedicle screws. Once the device is placed and secured to the screws, it is placed in ratchet position and distracted to obtain maximum correction. Once the adequate correction is obtained, the device is placed in locked position. No fusion is performed. Final confirmatory anteroposterior and lateral fluoroscopic images are taken (Figs. 15–18).

Postoperative protocol
Two to 3 weeks after the surgery, patients are directed to perform 5 basic Schroth exercises

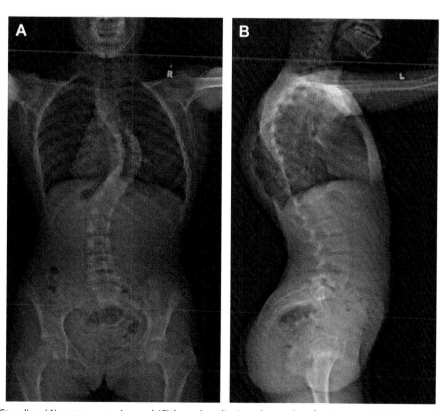

Fig. 15. Standing (A) posteroanterior and (B) lateral scoliosis radiographs of a 14-year-old, Risser 2 girl with 47° scoliosis and 40° of thoracic kyphosis.

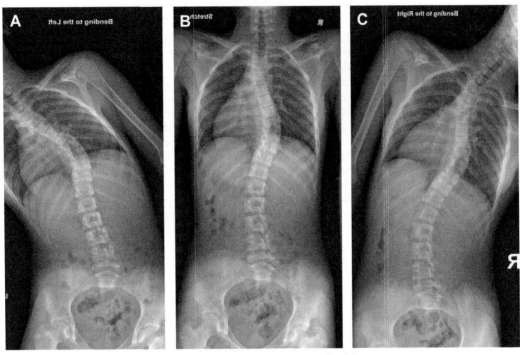

Fig. 16. (A–C) Bending and stretch radiographs demonstrating curve flexibility.

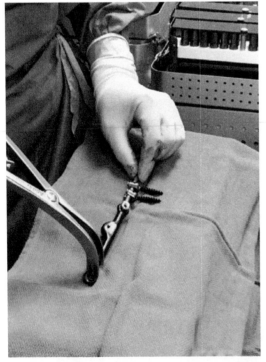

Fig. 17. Intraoperative picture showing assembly of the device and testing of the distraction mechanism before insertion. (*Courtesy of* ApiFix, Ltd, Misgav, Israel.)

that enable gradual elongation of the ratchet mechanism leading to a reduction of the spinal curve. These exercises consist of a hand hanging from a bar or door, lateral bending maneuvers while standing or sitting, and side stretching while lying on the side over a firm roll. The patient is instructed to perform the exercises for 30 minutes on a daily basis. Exercises are continued for 3 months after surgery.

Review of the literature
A biomechanical study by Holewijn and colleagues[55] demonstrated that the spinal range of motion of the bridged segments after spinal instrumentation with the posterior concave periapical nonfusion distraction device is partially diminished and adjacent segment biomechanics were not significantly altered. According to the authors, the periapical distraction device in free mode roughly halved spinal range of motion of flexion–extension (human 40.0% and porcine 55.9%), whereas lateral bending was only slightly affected (human 18.2% and porcine 17.9%) and axial rotation was unaffected. In comparison, the rigid pedicle screw–rod instrumentation resulted in a far greater decrease in the range of motion of flexion–extension (human 80.9% and porcine 94.0%), lateral bending (human 75.0% and porcine 92.2%), and axial rotation (human 71.3% and porcine 86.9%). The study

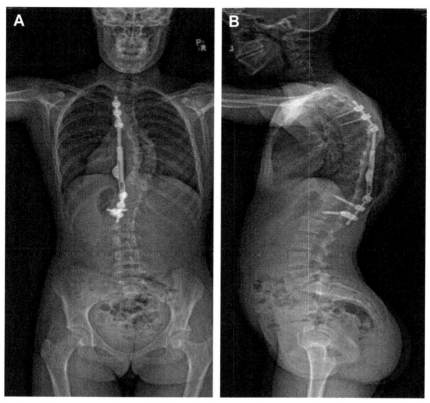

Fig. 18. Standing (*A*) posteroanterior and (*B*) lateral radiographs 6 months after the insertion of a posterior dynamic deformity correction device.

also reported that the periapical distraction device did not significantly affect adjacent segment motion. In contrast, after rigid pedicle screw–rod instrumentation, the range of motion of axial rotation decreased by 18.1% in the cranial adjacent segment of the human spines and increased by 23.9% in the caudal adjacent segment of the porcine spines.

Another biomechanical study by Arnin and colleagues[56] showed favorable static, fatigue, and wear resistance properties of the posterior dynamic deformity correction device. According to the authors, the system has 2 unique features: polyaxial joints at the rod–screw interface and a ceramic coating of the moving parts to overcome the challenges of wear and fatigue. Five biomechanical tests were performed: static compression to failure, fatigue loading per ASTM F 1717 with 5.5 mm screws for 10 MC at 5 Hz, wear assessment of full mechanism, wear test of the polyaxial joint under a 100-N load for 10 MC, and wear particle implantation in rabbits for 3 and 6 months. The study results demonstrated that the system failed through buckling of the rod with loads of greater than 3000 N. Dynamically, the system maintained

700 N for 10 million cycles with 5.5-mm screws. The maximum total steady-state wear rate was 0.074 mg per million cycles. Histologic evaluation of the particle injection sites indicated no difference in the local tissue response between the control and test articles. At 3 and 6 months after injection, there were neither adverse local effects nor systemic effects observed.

Because the ApiFix system is a novel less invasive short segment instrumentation, no long-term results have yet been published in the literature. Floman and colleagues[9] demonstrated the effectiveness of the periapical distraction device by reducing the Cobb angle from 43° to 53° to 22° to 33° in a series of 3 patients with a follow-up ranging from 6 months to 2 years. The authors stated that surgery takes less than 1 hour, blood loss is negligible, and no neurologic complications have been encountered. They reported that only 3 to 4 levels are instrumented, no fusion is performed, and the percentage of deformity correction is around 50%. No implant failures or unplanned returns to the operating room were encountered. Two weeks after surgery patients were pain free and were able to perform Schroth spinal

Table 4
Authors' preferred indications and contraindications for using the posterior dynamic deformity correction device

Authors' Preferred Indications	Authors' Preferred Contraindications
1. Cobb angle of 35°–60° (45°–60° if skeletally mature) 2. Flexible to ≤35° 3. Risser level 0–5 4. Age 11–18 y 5. Single thoracic/single lumbar or single thoracolumbar major curve	1. Stiff curve 2. Cobb angle of >60° 3. Double major/triple major curve

exercises and gradual elongation of the device was observed.

A recent retrospective, multicenter trial by Floman and colleagues[57] demonstrated the early results of the posterior dynamic deformity correction device for the treatment of AIS. Thirty-one patients with a minimum of 2 years of follow-up had a mean preoperative scoliosis of 49°, which improved to 34° with a correction of 32% at the final follow-up. All participating patients reported compliance with the exercise regimen and all patients were able to perform their exercises or other physical activities with no associated pain. Of the 31 patients, 5 underwent revision to an instrumented fusion. These revised patients all had preoperative scoliosis that was either greater than 60° or were not flexible preoperatively to 35° or less. Screw breakage, rod breakage, or ratchet problems were not encountered during the follow-up period. The investigators concluded that the device is a viable alternative to fusion and failed bracing for managing AIS and their current indication for the use of this device for AIS is less than 60° with flexibility to less than or equal to 35° (Table 4).

SUMMARY

Spinal fusion in young children for the treatment of EOS is not optimal because it limits growth and contributes to long-term lung compromise. Various types of growth-friendly spinal implants and newer technologies have been introduced in the past few years. Similarly, in AIS, fusion decreases spinal mobility and may lead to development of adjacent level disc degeneration. A variety of different new technologies have been developed for alternative surgical approaches that halt curve progression, while maintaining spinal mobility.

REFERENCES

1. Skaggs DL, Guillaume T, El-Hawary R, et al. Early onset scoliosis consensus statement, SRS growing spine committee, 2015. Spine Deform 2015;3(2):107.
2. Williams BA, Matsumoto H, McCalla DJ, et al. Development and initial validation of the classification of early-onset scoliosis (C-EOS). J Bone Joint Surg Am 2014;96(16):1359–67.
3. El-Hawary R, Akbarnia BA. Early onset scoliosis - time for consensus. Spine Deform 2015;3(2):105–6.
4. Skaggs DL, Akbarnia BA, Flynn JM, et al. A classification of growth friendly spine implants. J Pediatr Orthop 2014;34(3):260–74.
5. Bess S, Akbarnia BA, Thompson GH, et al. Complications of growing-rod treatment for early-onset scoliosis: analysis of one hundred and forty patients. J Bone Joint Surg Am 2010;92(15):2533–43.
6. Akbarnia BA, Cheung K, Noordeen H, et al. Next generation of growth-sparing techniques: preliminary clinical results of a magnetically controlled growing rod in 14 patients with early-onset scoliosis. Spine (Phila Pa 1976) 2013;38(8):665–70.
7. Ouellet J. Surgical technique: modern Luqué trolley, a self-growing rod technique. Clin Orthop Relat Res 2011;469(5):1356–67.
8. Hardesty CK, Huang RP, El-Hawary R, et al. Early-onset scoliosis: updated treatment techniques and results. Spine Deform 2018. https://doi.org/10.1016/j.jspd.2017.12.012.
9. Floman Y, Burnei G, Gavriliu S, et al. Surgical management of moderate adolescent idiopathic scoliosis with ApiFix®: a short peri-apical fixation followed by post-operative curve reduction with exercises. Scoliosis 2015;10(1):4.
10. Samdani AF, Ames RJ, Kimball JS, et al. Anterior vertebral body tethering for idiopathic scoliosis: two-year results. Spine (Phila Pa 1976) 2014;39(20):1688–93.
11. Weinstein SL, Dolan LA, Wright JG, et al. Effects of bracing in adolescents with idiopathic scoliosis. N Engl J Med 2013;369(16):1512–21.
12. Merenda L, Costello K, Santangelo AM, et al. Perceptions of self-image and physical appearance: conversations with typically developing youth and youth with idiopathic scoliosis. Orthop Nurs 2011;30(6):383–90.
13. Green DW, Lawhorne TW, Widmann RF, et al. Long-term magnetic resonance imaging follow-up demonstrates minimal transitional level lumbar disc degeneration after posterior spine fusion for adolescent idiopathic scoliosis. Spine (Phila Pa 1976) 2011;36(23):1948–54.

14. Danielsson AJ, Nachemson AL. Back pain and function 22 years after brace treatment for adolescent idiopathic scoliosis: a case-control study - Part I. Spine (Phila Pa 1976) 2003;28(18):2078–85.

15. Betz RR, Ranade A, Samdani AF, et al. Vertebral body stapling: a fusionless treatment option for a growing child with moderate idiopathic scoliosis. Spine (Phila Pa 1976) 2010;35(2):169–76.

16. Newton PO, Farnsworth CL, Faro FD, et al. Spinal growth modulation with an anterolateral flexible tether in an immature bovine model: disc health and motion preservation. Spine (Phila Pa 1976) 2008;33(7):724–33.

17. Newton PO, Fricka KB, Lee SS, et al. Asymmetrical flexible tethering of spine growth in an immature bovine model. Spine (Phila Pa 1976) 2002. https://doi.org/10.1097/00007632-200204010-00004.

10. Crawford CH, Lenke LG. Growth modulation by means of anterior tethering resulting in progressive correction of juvenile idiopathic scoliosis: a case report. J Bone Joint Surg Am 2010;92(1):202–9.

19. Dimeglio A, Canavese F, Charles P. Growth and adolescent idiopathic scoliosis. J Pediatr Orthop 2011;31(1):S28–36.

20. Dimeglio A, Canavese F. The growing spine: how spinal deformities influence normal spine and thoracic cage growth. Eur Spine J 2012;21(1):64–70.

21. Dimeglio A. Growth of the spine before age 5 years. J Pediatr Orthop B 1992;1(2):102–7.

22. Dimeglio A. Growth in Pediatric orthopaedics. J Pediatr Orthop 2001;21(4):549–55.

23. Dimeglio A, Canavese F. Progression or not progression? How to deal with adolescent idiopathic scoliosis during puberty. J Child Orthop 2013;7(1):43–9.

24. Campbell RM, Hell-Vocke AK. Growth of the thoracic spine in congenital scoliosis after expansion thoracoplasty. J Bone Joint Surg Am 2003;85(3):409–20.

25. Campbell RM, Smith MD, Mayes TC, et al. The characteristics of thoracic insufficiency syndrome. J Bone Joint Surg Am 2003;85(3):399–408. Available at: http://www.ncbi.nlm.nih.gov/pubmed/12637423. Accessed March 10, 2018.

26. Swank SM, Winter RB, Moe JH. Scoliosis and cor pulmonale. Spine (Phila Pa 1976) 1982;7(4):343–54.

27. Akbarnia BA, Campbell RM, Dimeglio A, et al. Fusionless procedures for the management of early-onset spine deformities in 2011: what do we know? J Child Orthop 2011;5(3):159–72.

28. Canavese F. Normal and abnormal spine and thoracic cage development. World J Orthop 2013;4(4):167.

29. Karol LA, Johnston C, Mladenov K, et al. Pulmonary function following early thoracic fusion in non-neuromuscular scoliosis. J Bone Joint Surg Am 2008;90(6):1272–81.

30. Canavese F, Dimeglio A, D'amato C, et al. Dorsal arthrodesis in prepubertal New Zealand white rabbits followed to skeletal maturity: effect on thoracic dimensions, spine growth and neural elements. Indian J Orthop 2010;44(1):14.

31. Gollogly S, Smith JT, White SK, et al. The volume of lung parenchyma as a function of age: a review of 1050 normal CT scans of the chest with three-dimensional volumetric reconstruction of the pulmonary system. Spine (Phila Pa 1976) 2004;29(18):2061–6.

32. Lonstein JE, Carlson JM. The prediction of curve progression in untreated idiopathic scoliosis during growth. J Bone Joint Surg Am 1984;66(7):1061–71.

33. Little DG, Song KM, Katz D, et al. Relationship of peak height velocity to other maturity indicators in idiopathic scoliosis in girls. J Bone Joint Surg Am 2000;82(5):685–93.

34. Little DG, Sussman MD. The Risser sign: a critical analysis. J Pediatr Orthop 1994;14(5):569–75.

35. Duval-Beaupére G. Remaining growth on the standing height and on the trunk after menarchis in girls. Rev Chir Orthop 1976;62:501.

36. Canavese F, Charles YP, Dimeglio A. Skeletal age assessment from elbow radiographs. Review of the literature. Chir Organi Mov 2008;92(1):1–6.

37. Song KM, Little DG. Peak height velocity as a maturity indicator for males with idiopathic scoliosis. J Pediatr Orthop 2000;20(3):286–8.

38. Sanders JO, Herring JA, Browne RH. Posterior arthrodesis and instrumentation in the immature (Risser-grade-0) spine in idiopathic scoliosis J Bone Joint Surg Am 1995;77(1):39–45. Available at: http://www.ncbi.nlm.nih.gov/pubmed/7822354. Accessed May 24, 2018.

39. Roberto RF, Lonstein JE, Winter RB, et al. Curve progression in Risser stage 0 or 1 patients after posterior spinal fusion for idiopathic scoliosis. J Pediatr Orthop 1997;17(6):718–25. Available at: http://www.ncbi.nlm.nih.gov/pubmed/9591972. Accessed May 24, 2018.

40. Wiesel WE. Spaceflight dynamics. Clin Ortop 1997;24(1):1–56. Available at: http://heyyou.allalla.com/pdf/spaceflight-dynamics-by-william-e-wiesel.pdf. Accessed May 24, 2018.

41. Hoppenfeld S, Lonner B, Murthy V, et al. The rib epiphysis and other growth centers as indicators of the end of spinal growth. Spine (Phila Pa 1976) 2004;29(1):47–50.

42. Herring JA, Tachdjian MO. Texas Scottish Rite Hospital for Children. Tachdjian's Pediatric Orthopaedics: From the Texas Scottish Rite Hospital for Children; 2015.

43. Takaso M, Moriya H, Kitahara H, et al. New remote-controlled growing-rod spinal instrumentation possibly applicable for scoliosis in young children. J Orthop Sci 1998;3(6):336–40.

44. Cheung JP, Bow C, Samartzis D, et al. Frequent small distractions with a magnetically controlled growing rod for early-onset scoliosisand avoidance of the law of diminishing returns. J Orthop Surg (Hong Kong) 2016;24(3):332–7.

45. Dannawi Z, Altaf F, Harshavardhana NS, et al. Early results of a remotely-operated magnetic growth rod in early-onset scoliosis. Bone Joint J 2013;95-B(1):75–80.

46. La Rosa G, Oggiano L, Ruzzini L. Magnetically controlled growing rods for the management of early-onset scoliosis: a preliminary report. J Pediatr Orthop 2017;37(2):79–85.

47. Rebollar ERL. The anatomic basis and development of segmental spinal instrumentation. Spine (Phila Pa 1976) 1982;7(3):256–9.

48. Ouellet JA, Ferland CE, Mehdian H. Growth-guided instrumentation: Luqué trolley. In: Akbarnia BA, Muharrem Y, Thompson GH, editors. The growing spine: management of spinal disorders in young children. 2nd edition. Berlin (Germany): Springer; 2015. p. 713–29.

49. Courvoisier A, Eid A, Bourgeois E, et al. Growth tethering devices for idiopathic scoliosis. Expert Rev Med Devices 2015;12(4):449–56.

50. Braun JT, Ogilvie JW, Akyuz E, et al. Creation of an experimental idiopathic-type scoliosis in an immature goat model using a flexible posterior asymmetric tether. Spine (Phila Pa 1976) 2006;31(13):1410–4.

51. Samdani AF, Ames RJ, Kimball JS, et al. Anterior vertebral body tethering for immature adolescent idiopathic scoliosis: one-year results on the first 32 patients. Eur Spine J 2015;24(7):1533–9.

52. Boudissa M, Eid A, Bourgeois E, et al. Early outcomes of spinal growth tethering for idiopathic scoliosis with a novel device: a prospective study with 2 years of follow-up. Childs Nerv Syst 2017; 33(5):813–8.

53. Danielsson AJ, Romberg K, Nachemson AL. Spinal range of motion, muscle endurance, and back pain and function at least 20 years after fusion or brace treatment for adolescent idiopathic scoliosis: a case-control study. Spine (Phila Pa 1976) 2006; 31(3):275–83.

54. Asher MA, Burton DC. Adolescent idiopathic scoliosis: natural history and long term treatment effects. Scoliosis 2006;1(1):2.

55. Holewijn RM, de Kleuver M, van der Veen AJ, et al. A novel spinal implant for fusionless scoliosis correction: a biomechanical analysis of the motion preserving properties of a posterior periapical concave distraction device. Global Spine J 2017; 7(5):400–9.

56. Arnin U, El-hawary R, et al. Pre-clinical bench testing on a novel posterior dynamic deformity correction device for scoliosis. Accept Spine Deform 2018. [Epub ahead of print].

57. Floman Y, Aviv T, et al. Early results from a retrospective pilot study of a posterior dynamic deformity correction device for the treatment of adolescent idiopathic scoliosis. Accept Spine Deform. [Epub ahead of print].

New Technologies in Pediatric Deformity Correction

Christopher A. Iobst, MD

KEYWORDS

• Limb deformities • Limb lengthening • Technology • Digital radiographs • 3D printing

KEY POINTS

• New technologies are available to evaluate limb alignment with more precision and less radiation than ever before.
• With the advent of digital radiographs, It is no longer necessary to manually plan deformity correction surgery using tracing paper and scissors.
• A digital Greulich and Pyle atlas has been found to save time, improve workflow experience, and reduce reporting errors.
• The field of 3-D printing is being integrated into pediatric deformity correction in many new and innovative approaches.
• Hexapod software systems are available that calculate the deformity parameters for external fixation based on radiographs of the deformed bone.

INTRODUCTION

The ability to correct limb deformities is one of the core elements of pediatric orthopedics. The term, *orthopedics*, is derived from the Greek language and means straightening (*ortho*) children (*paidos*). New advances in the evaluation and management of children with limb alignment or limb length issues are constantly appearing. This review highlights some of the recent technologies that have been developed to improve the care of these children.

NEW TECHNOLOGIES IN IMAGING

In the growing child, serial radiographs are often required to evaluate a child's limb alignment. The ability to measure the anatomic parameters of the lower limb in 3-D is essential in the analysis, diagnosis, and preoperative planning of lower limb deformity. New technologies are available to help perform this process and with more precision and less radiation than ever before. A new imaging method, using low-dose digital stereoradiography, uses a biplanar x-ray system that allows for 3-D modeling of the lower limbs.[1–6] Unlike axial CT scanograms and MRI, it is capable of producing full-length, weight-bearing images without any magnification error. More importantly, the images are captured with substantially smaller doses of radiation than plain radiographs or CT scans. This is especially critical in pediatric patients who may need long leg radiographs multiple times a year. By imaging the patient in the standing position, this technique removes any postural abnormalities that may occur when patients lie supine. For patients who are unable to stand or for those who are unsteady in the standing position, however, CT scan is still the preferred option.

Disclosure: C.A. Iobst is a consultant with Orthofix, NuVasive, and Smith & Nephew. No financial support was received for this study.
Department of Orthopedic Surgery, Center for Limb Lengthening and Reconstruction, The Ohio State University, College of Medicine, Nationwide Children's Hospital, 700 Children's Drive, Suite T2E-A2700, Columbus, OH 43205, USA
E-mail address: christopher.iobst@nationwidechildrens.org

In addition to allowing the standard coronal and sagittal plane deformity analysis to be performed, the real value with this imaging technique is the ability to simultaneously assess the rotational (axial) plane alignment. Axial-plane deformities of the lower limbs are often overlooked but are known to contribute to knee disorders, such as patellofemoral instability. The optimal management of lower limb rotational malalignment requires accurate and reproducible measurements of femoral version and tibial torsion. CT scan has traditionally been used for the analysis of limb segment rotation but the reproducibility of the measurements is highly dependent on the identification of proper skeletal landmarks. Using the biplanar technology, Folinais and colleagues[5] demonstrated that torsion values measured correlated closely with CT values, without bias and with comparably satisfactory interobserver reproducibility. The combination of multiplanar capabilities with the dramatic decrease in radiation dose versus conventional radiography or CT imaging suggests this technology will become the new gold standard in the assessment of pediatric limb deformity.

NEW TECHNOLOGIES IN DEFORMITY ANALYSIS

With the advent of digital radiographs, it is no longer necessary to manually plan deformity correction surgery using tracing paper and scissors. There is now a proprietary application for tablets that allows the surgeon to perform intricate deformity analysis on uploaded digital radiographs.[7] The application also permits virtual surgery to be performed on the limb by trialing and manipulating different osteotomy sites until the ideal combination is identified. The application has been compared with the picture archiving and communication system (PACS) used in most hospitals and found just as accurate in making deformity measurements. The study also found that the application made the analysis process faster than PACS measurements and had the advantage of being portable.

Similarly, a proprietary PACS integrated software system has been developed that contain tools designated for measuring various pediatric orthopedic pathologies, including limb length and angular measurements.[8–10] Digital measurements using this system have been found reliable in terms of intraobserver and interobserver variability. The software allows presurgical planning by permitting the surgeon to analyze the deformity, determine the deformity apex, choose the placement of the proposed osteotomy, and rearrange the fragments into anatomic alignment. In addition, the proper internal or external fixation devices and their respective components can be chosen from a list in the software program. The implant can then be templated to the image preoperatively. This feature permits the size and orientation of the desired device to be predicted precisely according to an individual patient's anatomy. The digital plan can then serve as a printed preoperative plan that the surgeon can reference during the procedure. The benefits of preoperative digital planning in limb deformity patients include accurate implant sizing, improved realignment accuracy, decreased operative time, and the anticipation of challenges and the preparation of solutions by the surgeon. It also can be used as a teaching tool for students, residents, fellows, colleagues, and patients to help visually explain anticipated complex deformity corrections.

NEW TECHNOLOGIES IN BONE AGE ASSESSMENT

Another area where digital planning is evolving in pediatric deformity correction is in the analysis of bone age radiographs. An accurate determination of bone age is critical when deciding the timing of guided growth or epiphysiodesis. Multiple techniques for assessing skeletal maturity have been described, but the most widely accepted technique is that of Greulich and Pyle.[11] The manual nature of the Greulich and Pyle method requires reviewing images and text within a book, looking up data in a chart, and making basic calculations, which slow diagnostic workflow and introduce the possibility of both observer and mathematical errors. This manual process can be even more challenging for trainees or infrequent users in general practice. A digital Greulich and Pyle atlas has been developed that can be integrated into PACS.[12] It has been found to save time, improve workflow experience, and reduce reporting errors relative to the Greulich and Pyle atlas when integrated into an electronic workflow. There are also smartphone applications available that provide portable shorthand bone age calculation guides.[13] Based on the work by Heyworth and colleagues,[14] the application allows the user to calculate the bone age in seconds without the need for the atlas. An automated method for determining bone age has also recently been investigated.[15] It examines the borders of 13 bones (radius, ulna, and 11 short bones in fingers 1, 3, and 5) and an intrinsic bone age is calculated from parameters, such as shape scores, bone density scores, and features describing the texture of the fusion in the growth plate. The intrinsic bone age is then transformed into the Greulich and Pyle bone age. This automated bone age determination system has been validated in white children with short statures and precocious puberty. A radiation-free assessment of bone age using quantitative ultrasound has been studied.[16] This technique uses a commercially available portable machine that evaluates 3 independent measurements of the radius and ulna epiphyses, metacarpals, and phalanx. After entering the patient's gender, the device software generated a bone age by using an integrated conversion equation. The initial results were found highly reproducible and comparable to bone age assessed by x-ray–based methods. Finally, 2 recent studies used artificial intelligence to develop an automatic software system for bone age determination using a Greulich and Pyle method–based deep-learning technique.[17,18] The automatic software system estimated skeletal maturity with accuracy similar to that of an expert radiologist and seemed to enhance efficiency by reducing reading times without compromising the diagnostic accuracy compared with traditional evaluation methods.

NEW TECHNOLOGIES IN 3-D PRINTING

The field of 3-D printing is being integrated into pediatric deformity correction in many new and innovative approaches. 3-D printing techniques can be used in preoperative planning to provide a better understanding of complex anatomy or morphology. A process known as rapid prototyping is an advanced manufacturing technology that produces high-fidelity solid 3-D structures from virtual 3-D renderings processed from CT images.[19] For example, 3-D printing can accurately replicate the actual size and spatial geometry of a deformed bone to facilitate the planning of treatment. Burzyńska and colleagues[20] used a printed 3-D bone model to prepare Ilizarov circular external fixation that spatially matched the size of the bones and prospective bone deformity. 3-D printing of the deformity made it possible to plan and test the experimental insertion of Ilizarov wires and the half-pins in the optimal spatial arrangement on the 3-D model. It also permitted trial correction of the deformity with the possibility of assessing the precision and the degree of accuracy of correction of the spatial location of the hinges and distractors of the Ilizarov frame. In addition,

this technique provided an opportunity to improve the process of training surgeons in the use of the Ilizarov method. The investigators concluded the 3-D printed models of bone allowed more detailed design of the apparatus and provided an opportunity for surgeons to anticipate possible problems that might arise during the operative procedure. These opportunities could then potentially shorten the operative time, reduce the risk of complications, and decrease the duration of treatment, resulting in better outcomes and lower treatment costs.

There are also commercially available hand-held 3-D mobile scanners that capture the shape of a desired body part, such as a limb, and create a high-resolution exact replica that can be manipulated on a computer.[21] Instead of just providing a replica of the bone, the scanner's paired software can produce a 3-D model of the limb with its overlying soft tissue envelope. This complete limb can then be 3-D printed to assist with designing an external fixator that fits the anatomic contours of the patient. This technology is already being used to create customized prosthetic and orthotic devices for patients.

An intraoperative application of 3-D printing involves the creation of customized implants or surgical guides.[22–24] 3-D–planned corrective osteotomies are a promising technique in the treatment of complex limb deformity. This technique permits the surgeon to visualize the anatomy in full 3-D and to digitally plan the osteotomy preoperatively, taking multiple surgical approaches into account. 3-D–planned corrective osteotomies generally involve 3 steps. First, data are collected by obtaining a CT scan of the deformed bone and contralateral healthy bone. Second, virtual models are created of both bones. By superimposing the deformed bone on a mirrored version of the healthy contralateral side, the location and degree of deformity are determined. A virtual osteotomy is then proposed within the region of the deformity, which divides the bone in a proximal and distal part. The distal and proximal part of the deformed bone can be rotated and translated to match with the contralateral bone. Finally, the preoperative plan is translated to the patient during the actual surgery. In its simplest form, the virtual or physical 3-D models can be used to aid a surgeon's understanding and visualization of the planned osteotomy plane. Alternatively, synthetic templates can be produced that can be placed in the osteotomy gap and restore the original position of the deformed bone. Patient-specific surgical cutting guides and fixation plates are made to match the patients' anatomy and include drilling guides and 1 or more osteotomy slits. Finally, the corrected position can be secured with the use of preoperatively defined, patient-specific plates.

The most appropriate use of this technology is still being defined. Clinical scenarios that are difficult to assess and address with conventional planning, such as rotational deformities of the forearm, intra-articular deformities, or complex multilevel, multiplanar long bone deformities, seem to be situations where this approach would be most beneficial. Clinical studies of distal radius malunions and hip dysplasia have both reported good outcomes using this technique.[22,24] de Muinck Keizer and colleagues[22] used 3-D–planned corrective osteotomies and showed significant improvement to both functional and radiographic results in patients with a malunion of the distal radius. Zheng and colleagues[24] generated a template to match the proximal femur in 11 pediatric patients with hip dysplasia or femoral neck fractures. After the feasibility of the 3-D model operation was demonstrated preoperatively, the guide pins and the screws were inserted with the help of the template intraoperatively. The fracture or osteotomy was fixed using a unique locking compression pediatric hip plate. The investigators commented that the technology diminished intraoperative damage to the femoral neck epiphysis, decreased operation time, reduced intraoperative hemorrhage, and limited radiation exposure to patients and personnel during the surgery.

Taking the 3-D printing process one step further, Qiao and colleagues[25] developed the first 3-D printed customized external fixator for long bone fracture reduction and fixation. Using reconstructed 3-D images of the fracture, reduction of the fracture model was performed on the computer. An external fixator made of photosensitive resin was designed and printed based on the new positions of bones and pins after the fracture model was reduced (**Fig. 1**). Fracture reduction by the computer-aided customized external fixator was found easier to manipulate, more accurate, and less dependent on surgeon experience compared with the Ilizarov apparatus. The major shortcoming with this technique is the prolonged time necessary to fabricate the frame. Therefore, after insertion of the fixation pins, the patient must wait approximately 20 hours for the fixator to be assembled.

Despite recent advances in prosthetic technology for upper extremity amputees, these

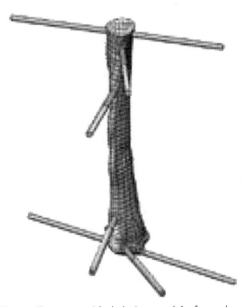

Fig. 1. Computer-aided design model of a reduced bone. (*From* Qiao F, Li D, Jin Z, et al. Application of 3D printed customized external fixator in fracture reduction. Injury 2015;46(6):1153; with permission.)

devices have had limited distribution in children. Most prostheses have been considered too expensive and/or too heavy to benefit a growing child. Children with upper limb differences, however, are ideal candidates for currently available 3-D–printed devices.[26] Print on-demand technology benefits pediatric prosthetic devices by making them customizable, affordable, and lightweight (**Fig. 2**). In addition, because children quickly outgrow prostheses, the low cost of 3-D printing makes repairs and upgrades affordable. Broken parts can be reprinted and replaced. The designs and color schemes are commonly tailored to a child's desires, and many children anecdotally report an increased social confidence having a personalized 3-D–printed hand that is colorful and fun. With the advent of plug-and-play desktop 3-D printers, anyone with access to the Internet can download available open-source design files and begin printing upper extremity prosthetic devices. The material cost of a printed and assembled hand is between $25 and $50. This affordability in prosthetic development is broadening access to prostheses around the world. This combination of qualities is sparking a resurgence of interest in children's prostheses and orthoses.

Although the field of 3-D printing seems to have unlimited potential in orthopedics, there are several concerns that remain. The first concern is how to regulate the output of

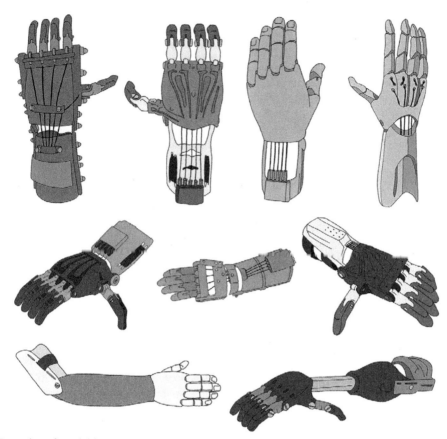

Fig. 2. Examples of available open-source hand models include (*left to right* and *top down*) Robohand, Cyborg Beast, Flexy Hand, K 1 Hand, Raptor Reloaded, Second Degree Hand, Osprey Hand, Limbitless Arm, and RIT Arm. These models are available through Web sites, such as ThingIverse (thingiverse.com) and the NIH 3D Print Exchange (3dprint.nih.gov). (*From* Tanaka KS, Lightdale-Miric N. Advances in 3D-printed pediatric prostheses for upper extremity differences. J Bone Joint Surg Am 2016;98(15):1324; with permission.)

3-D–printed products. The Food and Drug Administration is exploring ways of developing new standards that would take into account differences between traditional and 3-D printing manufacturing as well as the question of in-house manufacturing in hospitals. Second, the required time and cost of the techniques currently limit the convenience of 3-D printed materials. Preparation of patient-specific implants can take several weeks. In addition, 3-D printing technology requires access to materials and resources that are not available in many developing countries at this time. Third, to acquire the necessary data to construct the 3-D model, a patient must undergo a CT scan. This represents an additional radiation exposure to the patient. Finally, despite growing evidence showing the feasibility of rapid prototyping technology and its potential benefits in preparation for management of complex fractures, limb

deformity, and resident education, randomized clinical trials comparing the outcomes of this technique with conventional methods are lacking.

There are also several practical intraoperative limitations with 3-D printing that have been identified. First, when using 3-D–printed templates, a larger than normal surgical exposure may be necessary to position the guides. In some situations, the anatomy may limit the ability of the template to fit properly. There is also a concern that the increased soft tissue dissection may lead to wound complications in some patients. Second, maintaining reduction and compression of the osteotomy can be difficult. Although the reduction is facilitated by predrilled holes, the 3-D–printed guides are static, which may result is lack of compression or loss of reduction, especially in oblique osteotomies.

NEW TECHNOLOGIES IN LIMB LENGTHENING

The field of pediatric limb lengthening and limb deformity correction has recently undergone a substantial paradigm shift. Since the Ilizarov technique was first introduced to the Western world in the 1980s, external fixators have been used as the primary means to address limb deformity and limb length discrepancy. Because most pediatric patients with leg length discrepancy present with some combination of concomitant angular and/or rotational deformity, external fixators have traditionally been the only device capable of simultaneous multiplanar deformity. Despite possessing powerful capabilities, external fixators have recognized drawbacks, including patient discomfort, pin-track infections, and the overall bulkiness of the external construct. Consequently, surgeons have consistently been looking for alternative methods to perform limb lengthening. The concept of an intramedullary limb lengthening device has been considered since the 1980s. Being able to lengthen from inside the limb has always been an attractive idea because it alleviates the need for external pins, wires, or frames and conceivably makes the experience more comfortable for the patient. Unfortunately, the early attempts at intramedullary lengthening nail design produced devices that did not have reliable rate control, and the mechanism for lengthening was often painful to the patient.[27,28] Starting in 2012, a telescopic, titanium nail that is powered by magnets has been available to perform intramedullary lengthening. This device has proved reliable, accurate, and extremely comfortable for the patient.[29–31] The intramedullary lengthening method has many advantages: (1) a surgical technique that is familiar to most orthopedic surgeons; (2) the rate and rhythm of lengthening can be manipulated to the one-hundredth of a millimeter; and (3) the intramedullary implant protects the regenerate bone from deformation or fracture. Despite the many advantages and apparent simplicity of the technique, the surgeon must be cognizant that this is still limb lengthening. The same potential complications of joint contracture, joint dislocation, and neurovascular injury are still possible.

The success of the intramedullary lengthening implant has changed how deformity surgeons design treatment plans for their patients in 2 aspects. First, for pediatric patients with mild to moderate limb length discrepancies (ie, 3–5 cm), epiphysiodesis is no longer the only acceptable management option. If a patient wishes to conserve length and have a more predictable correction of the limb length discrepancy, it is reasonable to offer intramedullary lengthening instead of epiphysiodesis. Second, surgeons are looking to develop treatment plans for their patients that completely avoid the use of an external fixator. Although a patient with a limb length discrepancy and an angular or rotational deformity would previously require an external fixator, the new thought process is to try to correct everything using internal methods. For example, angular corrections can initially be performed using guided growth, plating, or rodding followed by subsequent intramedullary lengthening. For pediatric patients approaching skeletal maturity, intramedullary lengthening nails also can be used to simultaneously correct angular/rotational deformity and length using blocking screws.[32]

NEW TECHNOLOGIES IN EXTERNAL FIXATION

Although intramedullary limb lengthening nails have revolutionized the field of limb lengthening over the past 5 years, there are still situations where external fixators are necessary. Since the late 1990s, hexapod circular external fixators have been commercially available to perform multiplanar corrections. These devices are paired with a software program to help guide the surgeon through the deformity analysis and deformity correction process. Improvements to the software portion of the hexapod external fixation systems have been made. Traditionally, the surgeon would manually perform the deformity analysis and enter those parameters into the software. Now, there are hexapod software systems available that calculate the deformity parameters for the surgeon based on anteroposterior and lateral radiographs of the deformed bone. The surgeon uploads the images into the software and marks key landmarks on each image, which allows the software to analyze the deformity. The surgeon can then place an osteotomy line at various positions and the software determines the optimal amount of angular, translational, and axial correction necessary to achieve the desired result. The surgeon can also determine the size, level of attachment, and orientation of the hexapod rings using the software to create a comprehensive preoperative plan. New software also has the ability to account for imperfect frame mounting by the surgeon. At the end of the case, the surgeon can simply input that the frame was angled or rotated and the computer makes the adjustments without having to change the deformity or mounting parameters. Another improvement in the software is the dampening of the bone movement that occurs during the correction.[33] Older software brought the bone ends from point A to point B by in a series of spiral movements until the bone ends reached their final destination. Newer software models dampen the amount of bone spiraling that occurs and move the bone ends to the final destination in more of a straight line. This decreased bone travel may help to improve healing times. New software packages now allow the surgeon multiple options to control the correction process. The surgeon can choose to move the bone in millimeters per day, degrees of angulation, degrees of rotation, or simply by the desired number of days. The software can also divide the program into 2 independent components running at different rates. For example, if a surgeon wants to distract the bone fragments a certain amount before attempting angular correction, the correction program can be devised to perform 1 mm per day lengthening and then, on completion of the distraction, start the angular correction at 2° per day. There is no longer any need to create separate programs for each of these way points. Finally, in a world dominated by smartphones, it is only natural that the hexapod software should be compatible with the phones. Applications now exist where a patient's prescription can be loaded into a phone. The patient can follow the progress of the daily adjustments and receive reminders on a phone when it is time to perform the adjustments. The surgeon can also choose to monitor a patient's progress remotely and send inspirational or educational messages to the patient.

Advances in the hexapod hardware have also been seen. Radiolucent circular rings made of braided carbon fiber are lighter and improve the visualization of the joint line, the fracture site or the osteotomy site that otherwise would be obscured by metal rings. Modular rings are available that allow the surgeon to transition from a full ring to a 5/8 ring or vice versa as needed. Another new ring design has slots instead of discrete holes for placement of the half-pin and wire fixation elements. This potentially increases the fixation options for the surgeon and improves the versatility of the system. Struts have also undergone some major design changes. Some ring fixators now have struts that attach to the outside of the rings rather than underneath the rings. This increases

the amount of space available for rotation inside the ring as well as the space available for placement of the fixation elements between the struts and the rings.[34] Struts are also available with a combination of acute and gradual correction in 1 element. This helps limit the number of strut changes necessary during a given deformity correction. Having fewer strut changes saves time for health care providers in clinics and saves cost to patients. The combination of acute and gradual correction in one strut also helps limit the inventory of struts needed.

Struts can now be adjusted in increments less than 1 mm. Depending on the type of strut, the adjustments can be as small as 0.25 mm or 0.5 mm. Struts are also designed with knobs to prevent inadvertent adjustments from occurring when patients moves their limbs around in bed. Some struts have a ball-and-socket design that allows the frame to be rigid. The rings can even be placed very close together without losing stability, which can be important in short pediatric limbs with large deformities.[35] Some strut designs allow controlled dynamization to be performed anywhere from 1 mm to 5 mm, which can be helpful in patients with fractures. Commercially available axial dynamization modules can be added to threaded rods to allow 0.5-mm to 3.5-mm axial micromovement when the surgeon wants to add controlled dynamization to the patient. Regarding fixation elements, hydroxyapatite coating is now available on Ilizarov wires and iodine-supported half-pins have also been developed as a means of decreasing pin-track infections.[36]

FUTURE TECHNOLOGY

The combination of gene therapy and tissue engineered scaffolds is a promising multidisciplinary approach to bone repair with significant clinical potential. Alluri and colleagues[37] loaded human adipose-derived stem cells that were virally transduced to produce BMP-2 onto a 3-D printed scaffold comprised of hyperelastic "bone." This novel, surgically friendly composite material has promising clinical potential to treat skeletal defects due to its desirable combination of properties. Mechanically, the composite is readily malleable yet retains biomechanical properties similar to that of cortical bone. Biologically, the composite is a combination of a highly osteoconductive 3-D printed scaffold combined that delivers transduced human cells that overexpress a highly osteoinductive signal.

REFERENCES

1. Demzik AL, Alvi HM, Delagrammaticas DE, et al. Inter-rater and intra-rater repeatability and reliability of EOS 3-dimensional imaging analysis software. J Arthroplasty 2016;31:1091–5.

2. Gaumétoua E, Quijanob S, Ilharrebordea B, et al. EOS analysis of lower extremity segmental torsion in children and young adults. Orthop Traumatol Surg Res 2014;100:147–51.

3. Guenouna B, Zadegan F, Aim F, et al. Reliability of a new method for lower-extremity measurements based on stereoradiographic three-dimensional reconstruction. Orthop Traumatol Surg Res 2012; 98:506–13.

4. Wybier M, Bossard P. Musculoskeletal imaging in progress: the EOS imaging system. Joint Bone Spine 2013;80:238–43.

5. Folinais D, Thelen P, Delin C, et al. Measuring femoral and rotational alignment: EOS system versus computed tomography. Orthop Traumatol Surg Res 2013;99:509–16.

6. Delin C, Silvera S, Bassinet C, et al. Ionizing radiation doses during lower limb torsion and anteversion measurements by EOS stereoradiography and computed tomography. Eur J Radiol 2014;83: 371–7.

7. Whitaker AT, Gesheff MG, Jauregui JJ, et al. Comparison of PACS and Bone Ninja mobile application for assessment of lower extremity limb length discrepancy and alignment. J Child Orthop 2016; 10:439–43.

8. Segev E, Hemo Y, Wientroub S, et al. Intra- and interobserver reliability analysis of digital radiographic measurements for pediatric orthopedic parameters using a novel PACS integrated computer software program. J Child Orthop 2010;4:331–41.

9. Siddiqui NA, Lamm BM. Digital planning for foot and ankle deformity correction: evans osteotomy. J Foot Ankle Surg 2014;53:700–5.

10. Atesok K, Galos D, Jazrawi LM, et al. Preoperative planning in orthopaedic surgery current practice and evolving applications. Bull Hosp Joint Dis 2015;73:257–68.

11. Greulich WW, Pyle SI. Radiographic atlas of skeletal development of the hand and wrist. 2nd edition. Stanford (CA): Stanford University Press; 1959.

12. Bunch PM, Altes TA, McIlhenny J, et al. Skeletal development of the hand and wrist: digital bone age companion—a suitable alternative to the Greulich and Pyle atlas for bone age assessment? Skeletal Radiol 2017;46:785–93. Available at: http://www.life-bridgehealth.org/RIAO/InternationalCenterforLimbLengthening2.aspx. Accessed August 30, 2018.

13. Multiplier. International Center for Limb Lengthening Rubin Institute for Advanced Orthopedics Sinai Hospital of Baltimore.

14. Heyworth BE, Osei DA, Fabricant PD, et al. The shorthand bone age assessment: a simpler alternative to current methods. J Pediatr Orthop 2013;33: 569–74.

15. Satoh M. Bone age: assessment methods and clinical applications. Clin Pediatr Endocrinol 2015;24: 143–52.

16. Rachmiel M, Naugolni L, Mazor-Aronovitch K, et al. Bone age assessments by quantitative ultrasound (SonicBone) and hand X-ray based methods are comparable. Isr Med Assoc 2017;19:533–8.

17. Kim JR, Shim WH, Yoon HM, et al. Computerized bone age estimation using deep learning based program: evaluation of the accuracy and efficiency. Am J Roentgenol 2017;209:1374–80.

18. Larson DB, Chen MC, Lungren MP, et al. Performance of a deep-learning neural network model in assessing skeletal maturity on pediatric hand radiographs. Radiology 2018;287:313–22.

19. Martelli N, Serrano C, van den Brink H, et al. Advantages and disadvantages of 3-dimensional printing in surgery: a systematic review. Surgery 2016;159: 1485–500.

20. Burzyńska K, Morasiewicz P, Filipiak J. The use of 3D printing technology in the ilizarov method treatment: pilot study. Adv Clin Exp Med 2016; 25:1157–63.

21. 3D Acanners. Artec Europe. Available at: https://www.artec3d.com. Accessed August 30, 2018.

22. de Muinck Keizer RJO, Lechner KM, Mulders MAM, et al. Three-dimensional virtual planning of corrective osteotomies of distal radius malunions: a systematic review and meta-analysis. Strategies Trauma Limb Reconstr 2017;12:77–89.

23. Hoekstra H, Rosseels W, Sermon A, et al. Corrective limb osteotomy using patient specific 3D-printed guides: a technical note. Injury 2016;47: 2375–80.

24. Zheng P, Yao Q, Xu P, et al. Application of computer-aided design and 3D-printed navigation template in Locking Compression Pediatric Hip Plate™ placement for pediatric hip disease. Int J Comput Assist Radiol Surg 2017;12:865–71.

25. Qiao F, Li D, Jin Z, et al. Application of 3D printed customized external fixator in fracture reduction. Injury 2015;46:1150–5.

26. Tanaka KS, Lightdale-Miric N. Advances in 3D-printed pediatric prostheses for upper extremity differences. J Bone Joint Surg Am 2016;98:1320–6.

27. Guichet JM, Deromedis B, Donnan LT, et al. Gradual femoral lengthening with the Albizzia intramedullary nail. J Bone Joint Surg Am 2003; 85:838–48.

28. Lee DH, Ryu KJ, Song HR, et al. Complications of the intramedullary skeletal kinetic distractor in distraction osteogenesis. Clin Orthop Relat Res 2014;472:3852–9.

29. Kirane YM, Fragomen AT, Rozbruch SR. Precision of the Precice internal bone lengthening nail. Clin Orthop Rel Res 2014;472:3869–78.
30. Herzenberg J, Standard S, Conway J, et al. Satisfaction of patients who have undergone lengthening with both internal and external fixation: a comparison study. LLRS 2013 Annual Meeting, New York, July 19-20.
31. Paley D. Precice intramedullary limb lengthening system. Expert Rev Med Devices 2015;12(3): 231–49.
32. Iobst CA, Rozbruch SR, Nelson S, et al. Simultaneous acute femoral deformity correction and gradual limb lengthening using a retrograde femoral nail. technique and clinical results. J Am Acad Orthop Surg 2018;26:241–50.
33. Cherkashin A. Mathematical modeling for the evaluation of hexapod frames stability and correction path. Limb Lengthening and Reconstruction Society 25th Annual Scientific Meeting, Charleston, SC, July 22, 2016.
34. Iobst CA, Cherkashin A, Samchukov M. Comparison of hexapod frame systems. JLLR 2016;2(1): 29–34.
35. Samchukov M, Chiaramonti B, Leonchuk S, et al. Comparative conformational instability of different hexapod frames. JLLR 2015;1(Suppl. 1):S13.
36. Shirai T, Watanabe K, Matsubara H, et al. Prevention of pin tract infection with iodine-supported titanium pins. J Orthop Sci 2014;19: 598–602.
37. Alluri R, Jakus A, Bougioukli S, et al. 3D printed hyperelastic "bone" scaffolds and regional gene therapy: a novel approach to bone healing. J Biomed Mater Res A 2018;106A: 1104–10.

Hand and Wrist

Emerging Technologies in Upper Extremity Surgery

Polyvinyl Alcohol Hydrogel Implant for Thumb Carpometacarpal Arthroplasty and Processed Nerve Allograft and Nerve Conduit for Digital Nerve Repairs

William J. Weller, MD

KEYWORDS

- Thumb carpometacarpal arthroplasty • Polyvinyl alcohol hydrogel implant
- Processed nerve allograft • Nerve conduit • Digital nerve repair

---

KEY POINTS

- New and developing technology in the field of upper extremity surgery offers promise of improved outcomes.
- Polyvinyl alcohol hydrogel implants may provide improved treatment of thumb carpometacarpal arthroplasty for Eaton stage II or stage III arthritis.
- Current data suggest that processed nerve allografts are indicated for digital nerve gaps of 10 mm or more, with high rates of sensory recovery.
- Nerve conduits seem indicated for digital nerve gaps of less than 10 mm.
- Larger studies with longer follow-up are needed to clarify indications, outcomes, and safety of these technologies.

POLYVINYL ALCOHOL HYDROGEL IMPLANT FOR THUMB CARPOMETACARPAL ARTHROPLASTY

Background

The polyvinyl alcohol hydrogel (PVA-H) implant (Fig. 1) is one of the most recent developments in hand surgery for treating thumb carpometacarpal (CMC) osteoarthritis. Although it is new in its application in hand surgery, this biomaterial has been and is currently used in soft contact lenses, first metatarsophalangeal joint replacement, artificial vitreous solution, tissue adhesion barriers, artificial tears, synthetic articular surface replacement in the knee, and close-contact packaging for food products.[1] The implant is an organic polymer-based biomaterial composed of 40% polyvinyl alcohol and saline.[1,2] It is produced by partial or full hydrolysis of acetate to remove the acetate groups. Next the polymer is cross-linked with freezing and thawing cycles, thus producing structural stability for the implant in aqueous solutions.[3,4] The result is a soft hydrogel that has favorable biochemical and wear characteristics, such as low protein adsorption, low cell adhesion properties, and wear particulate generation that causes less inflammation than ultra-high-molecular-weight polyethylene (UHMWPE) particulates.[1,5] Furthermore, PVA-H implants can be manufactured to display tensile strength and compressive modulus similar to the ranges demonstrated by native cartilage.[1,4] They have been shown to exhibit biphasic mechanical

---

Department of Orthopaedic Surgery and Biomedical Engineering, University of Tennessee-Campbell Clinic, 1211 Union Avenue, Suite 510, Memphis, TN 38104, USA
E-mail address: williamjacobweller@gmail.com

Orthop Clin N Am 50 (2019) 87–93
https://doi.org/10.1016/j.ocl.2018.08.011

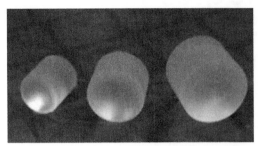

Fig. 1. PVA-H implants for thumb CMC arthroplasty. (*From* Taleb C, Berner S, Mantovani Ruggiero G. First metacarpal resurfacing with polyvinyl alcohol implant in rhizarthrosis: preliminary study. Chir Main 2014;33(3):191; with permission.)

properties through rapid water loss, with initial compressive loading and resorption of water with off-loading. The PVA-H biomaterial also exhibits a fluid film with loading, thus producing a coefficient of friction in the range of 0.04 to 0.07, which is comparable to native cartilage (typical range of native cartilage <0.01–0.05, cobalt chrome on UHMWPE 0.05–0.15).[1,4–7]

Indications

The primary indication for this procedure is thumb CMC arthritis with either Eaton stage II or stage III degenerative changes (**Fig. 2**). Eaton stage IV arthritis is a contraindication to implantation of this device, because it affects only the articulating surface of the first metacarpal and trapezium and does not replace the scaphoid-trapezium-trapezoid articulations. Eaton stage I is better treated with volar beak reconstruction or first metacarpal base osteotomy. Other contraindications include active infection, patients younger than 18 years of age, poor trapezial, or first metacarpal bone stock, and severe joint instability.[2,8,9]

Clinical Outcomes

The data on clinical use of PVA-H implants for thumb CMC arthroplasty are limited, with only 1 published report at this point. This 2014 study is a case series of 7 patients with either Eaton stage II or stage III basilar thumb arthritis. At a mean short-term follow-up of 30 months, no complications were noted and Disabilities of the Arm, Shoulder and Hand (DASH) scores improved from 93/100 (range 78–100) preoperatively to 40/100 (range 0–65) at last follow-up. Mean visual analog scores (VAS) also improved from 8/10 (range 7–10) preoperatively to 2/10 (range 0–5) postoperatively. The mean grip strength went from 11 kg (range 10–22 kg) to 20 kg (range 9–33 kg), and mean pinch

improved from 2.4 kg (range 1.5–3 kg) to 4.6 kg (range 2–6 kg). Radiographic monitoring showed no dislocation or osteolysis, and MRI showed no inflammatory reaction to the implant.[2]

Although this small case series shows some compelling findings, the multicenter GRIP study recently completed in Canada and the United Kingdom will be published sometime later this year. The GRIP study of 44 patients with 1-year follow-up will be the first prospective feasibility study published on the PVA-hydrogel implant for thumb arthroplasty. The objectives of this study, as stated on the United States clinical trials governmental Web site, were to evaluate the safety and effectiveness of Cartiva synthetic cartilage implant (SCI) for CMC in terms of pain relief and improvement of joint function in patients with first CMC osteoarthritis and to evaluate Cartiva SCI for CMC device performance to establish the parameters for a pivotal trial. Follow-up visits occurred at 5 time points after the surgical procedure: 14 days, 42 days, 90 days, 180 days, and 1 year. The primary outcome measure was pain as measured by the VAS.[8] In addition to the first GRIP study, the follow-up GRIP 2 began patient enrollment here in the United States and in the United Kingdom in December of 2017. The GRIP 2 study will be a prospective noninferiority study comparing the Cartiva SCI for CMC device with ligament reconstruction and tendon interposition (LRTI). The primary outcomes measured will be VAS, quick DASH, radiographs, and safety in terms of requiring secondary procedures.[9] The data provided from these 2 studies will shed much needed light on the clinical usefulness of this device in addressing thumb CMC arthritis.

Although long-term data on PVA-H implant use in the thumb CMC are lacking, 5-year data on its use in first MTP arthroplasty were reported in 2016. The study by Daniels and colleagues[10] included 29 patients of whom only 2 were lost to follow-up at 5 years. This represents the first 43% of study patients to reach 5-year follow-up after PVA-H arthroplasty. The results at 5 years showed 96% implant survivorship, with only 1 implant converted to fusion, significantly improved standardized functional scores compared with preoperative baselines, and mean VAS scores of 5.7 on a 100-point scale. Additionally, 23 of the 27 patients had radiographic follow-up with no changes in implant position, loosening, osteolysis, subsidence, or implant wear. The only radiographic changes noted were small cysts in the proximal phalanx that did not require intervention. Another,

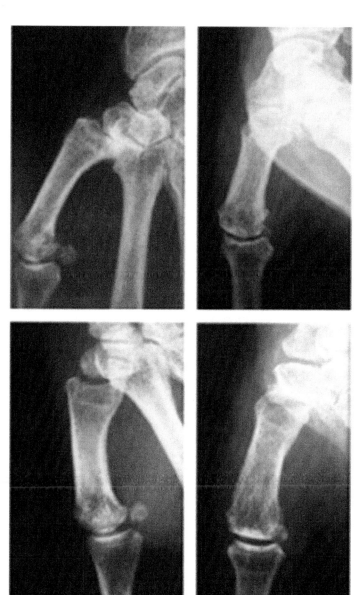

Fig. 2. A 67-year-old woman with Littler stage II osteoarthritis of the right thumb. (*Top*) Preoperative radiographs; (*bottom*) 16 months after surgery. The space created by the implant is visible on the lateral view. (*From* Taleb C, Berner S, Mantovani Ruggiero G. First metacarpal resurfacing with polyvinyl alcohol implant in rhizarthrosis: preliminary study. Chir Main 2014;33(3):192; with permission.)

larger study comparing 147 PVA-H first MTP implants to 47 first MTP fusions with 2-year follow-up showed an 11% secondary surgery rate for the PVA-H implants.[11] These studies provide the early logical support for the use of this implant in thumb CMC arthroplasty; however, further studies are needed to support its use beyond the experimental realm.

Summary

PVA-H implant for thumb CMC arthroplasty is an emerging technology that warrants further investigation. Its bioinert characteristics and biomechanics similar to cartilage make it a desirable material for use in joint reconstruction. Furthermore, it offers an alternative option for younger patients with Eaton stage II or stage III osteoarthritis because it can potentially provide good pain relief while removing minimal bone stock. The longevity of the implant is unclear; however, LRTI is still possible after PVA-H arthroplasty because of its minimal bone resection. The upcoming publication of the GRIP 1 study and later publication of the GRIP 2 study will provide further insight into this device regarding its durability, outcomes, and safety.

PROCESSED NERVE ALLOGRAFT AND NERVE CONDUIT USE IN DIGITAL NERVE REPAIR

Cadaver nerve allografts have been increasingly used in hand surgery since 2010 after the Food and Drug Administration approved the first processed nerve allograft (PNA), Avance Nerve Graft (AxoGen, Alachua, Florida), for use in the United States. Since that time, the clinical use of PNA has continued to expand and be studied. Nerve conduit use, however, preceded PNA by approximately 10 years and often was compared with direct repair of nerves, with only moderate improvement of outcomes at varying nerve gap lengths. As PNA use continued to grow, it was initially unclear as to when PNA was indicated over nerve conduits. Only in the past few years have studies begun to elucidate the limits of and best indications for conduits versus PNA. The establishment of the Retrospective Study of Advance Nerve Graft Utilization, Evaluations and Outcomes in Peripheral Nerve Injury Repair (RANGER) database and Comparative Study of Hollow Nerve Conduit and Advance Nerve Graft Evaluation Recovery Outcomes of the Nerve Repair in the Hand (CHANGE) study, both done in part with the developer, AxoGen Incorporated, have been largely responsible for the current data comparing PNA to nerve conduits.

Background: Processed Nerve Allograft

PNA is created at an American Association of Tissue Banks–accredited facility from harvested cadaver nerves of 1 mm in diameter up to 5 mm in diameter. The longest PNA approved by the Food and Drug Administration is 70 mm, but these can be linked in series, or daisy-chained, to create longer nerve allografts when needed.[12] The most important aspects of processing nerve allograft are removal of the immunogenic cells and cellular debris, while still maintaining the nerve allograft ultrastructure made up of extracellular matrix proteins and basal lamina. The more the allograft is processed to rid it of Schwann cells, myelin, and other major histocompatibility–containing elements, the less likely an immune response will occur during regrowth of the axons down the lumen of the allograft. Too much processing or deep freezing, however, can lead to disruption of the allograft ultrastructure and impede nerve regrowth inside the allograft.[13] Additionally, removal of the Schwann cells, although necessary to prevent immune rejection, robs the PNA of signaling cues that can be beneficial for axon regeneration. At the most basic level the PNA should retain the basal lamina, which is requisite for distal axon sprouting and nerve regrowth.[13–20]

The exact method by which vendors produce PNA is proprietary and differs depending on the developer; however, the process generally uses chemical detergents, radiation, enzymes such as elastase or chondroitinase, and freezing.[12,15–21] After the extensive processing is complete, the allograft is cryopreserved at 4°C and then thawed until just before implantation. On the horizon are loading nerve growth factor (NGF) additives to the PNA. In a recent in vitro study, Thayer and colleagues preloaded rat PNA with NGF and were able to show significant retention of half the NGF in the PNA after day 1 and then up to 15% NGF retention at 21 days. The investigators also compared processing protocols and found better maintenance of PNA ultrastructure and retention of NGF with the specific processing described by Sondell and colleagues.[19] The addition of these growth factors and other chemical mediators to PNA may be the pathway to improving the outcomes of PNA grafting of larger nerve defects.

Background: Nerve Conduits

Nerve conduits are derived from numerous substrates, including processed porcine intestinal submucosa, polyglycolic acid, processed bovine based type I collagen, autologous veins, and polycaprolactone.[22–27] They range in diameter from 1.5 mm to 7 mm and in lengths to 15 mm. The logic behind a nerve conduit is that it creates a semipermeable enclosed environment between the nerve ends thus preventing intrusion of fibroblasts between the sprouting axons while allowing diffusion of glucose, oxygen, and growth factors into that enclosed environment. It also bridges gaps, thus allowing for a more tension-free repair, and keeps neurotrophic factors within the closed environment between the nerve ends. The conduit additionally allows fibrin matrix accumulation, which is believed to act as the scaffold on which the axons grow while bridging the gap.[22,27] The number of axons that bridge the gap, however, is directly proportional to the narrowest diameter of the fibrin matrix within the conduit. As a result, the regenerating nerve tends to take on an hourglass appearance as the fibrin tends to contract as it matures, potentially limiting the number of bridging axons reaching the distal native nerve end.[27] Additionally, the conduits are designed to be degraded by the body over time, but some reports have shown retention of parts of the conduit at the coaptation site with scarring, inflammatory reaction, and wound fistulas. Most of these complications have been associated with the polycaprolactone-derived conduit, which is no longer recommended.[28,29] Despite complications with mainly the polycaprolactone based conduits, there is still a safe role for the other nonpolycaprolactone-based conduits in peripheral nerve repair. Autologous veins also have been used and, in a well-designed prospective randomized study, have proven equivalent in terms of static 2-point discrimination (S2PD) recovery and cost compared with conduits.[26]

Indications
Over the past 5 years studies have begun to define the digital nerve gap lengths in which conduits perform well and gap lengths that are better served with PNA. Before determination of the nerve gap, the traumatized nerve tissue should be adequately débrided back to pouting fascicles with good punctate bleeding noted within the perineural architecture with the tourniquet released. Additionally, the gap should be determined to account for maximal joint range of motion that will be allowed during the early rehabilitation process. Once the gap is determined with those aspects in mind, the surgeon can then choose to use a conduit or a PNA.[27,30] The current general consensus from the available data supports use of nerve conduits in nerve gaps of less than 10 mm. Conversely, the use of PNA is best indicated for nerve gaps of 10 mm or more. The upper limit of the nerve gap for which PNA is best indicated, however, is unknown based on current data.[27]

Clinical Outcomes of Processed Nerve Allograft
The AxoGen-sponsored CHANGE study was one of the first to publish results of a double-blind, prospective, multicenter, randomized study comparing PNA to bovine type I collagen-based hollow nerve conduits. The average gap length before repair was 12 mm ± 4 mm (5–20 mm range). Their results were promising, with the PNA having a significantly better S2PD of 5 mm ± 1 mm compared with 8 mm ± 5 mm for nerve conduit at 12 months postoperative. Although the patient numbers were low (PNA n = 6, conduit n = 9) because of attrition, for patients who reached 12-month follow-up the final results showed 100% of PNA recovered at least S3+ Medical Research Council classification (MRCC) of sensory function compared with 75% of the conduits attaining S3+ function. Additionally, return to S4 level for patients reaching 12-month follow-up was 80% in the PNA group

compared with 50% in the conduit cohort; however, this did not reach statistical significance.[22]

The findings of the CHANGE study indicating PNA for nerve gaps of more 10 mm are supported by additional publications. A case series of 8 digital nerves with PNA reconstruction of mean nerve gaps of 21 mm (range 5–30 mm) reported return of S2PD to S4 function in all.[31] Another small case series of 5 digital nerve defects of 23 mm (range 18–28 mm) reconstructed with PNA reported that 4 patients recovered S2PD of S4 function with the lone outlier having S2PD of 7 mm.[32] Taras and colleagues[33] published a larger prospective PNA study of 18 digital nerve injuries with an average gap length of 11 mm (range 5–30 mm). The investigators developed their own classification system for outcomes, which makes it difficult to compare outcomes to other published metrics. By extrapolating their S2PD results to MRCC for the sake of comparison, however, this study found that 12 of the 18 patients recovered S3+ function and an additional 6 patients recovered S4 function.

Another major study evaluating PNA was the first RANGER database study published in 2012 by Cho and colleagues.[34] This multicenter retrospective study looked at 71 PNA reconstructions for mixed, motor, and sensory nerves, 35 of which were digital nerve reconstructions. The mean digital nerve gap length was 19 mm (range 5–50 mm), and 31 patients (89%) with digital nerve PNA reconstructions achieved S3 or S4 sensory function, or what they defined as "meaningful recovery on the MRCC scale." Additionally, 100% of nerve gaps < 15 mm achieved S3 sensory function. However when the authors assessed the data for return of just S3+ function, it was found that still 76% of patients achieved this level of sensory return in digital nerve PNA reconstruction with a mean gap length of 19 mm.

The follow-up RANGER database study published in 2016 comprised 50 digital nerve injuries with an average gap length of 35 mm (range 27–50). To evaluate the outcomes of PNA at larger gap lengths, the investigators queried the database for gaps of more than 25 mm. They reported that 43 (86%) reconstructions achieved S3 function or greater, with 32 (64%) reconstructions achieving S3+ or S4 levels of recovery. These values were found consistent independent of the gap range up to 50 mm. They reported no adverse events and found the outcomes comparable with historical studies for autografting.[35]

Clinical Outcomes of Nerve Conduits
Prior to the CHANGE study, conduits often were compared with direct nerve repair. In one of the

earliest studies on conduits, Weber and colleagues[36] found that 91% of polyglycolic acid conduit repairs regained S4 MRCC function compared with only 49% of direct digital nerve repairs achieving S4 MRCC in gap lengths less than 4 mm. This early study suggested that conduits are best indicated for smaller nerve gaps. A follow-up study in 2011 by Taras and colleagues[37] reported that 55% of patients recovered S4 function with a mean gap length of 12 mm with nerve conduit repair of digital nerves. Another study of conduit use in digital nerve gaps reported that 63% of patients obtained at least S3+ sensory function with mean gap lengths of 12 mm.[38] As researchers began to realize that outcomes varied widely with conduit use in larger nerve gaps, and with PNA emerging as a potential answer for larger nerve gaps, recommendations for the use of conduits continued but at smaller gap lengths. Schmauss and colleagues[39] in 2014 ultimately showed the usefulness of conduits for nerve gaps of less than 10 mm. Safa and Buncke[27] and Isaacs[30] provide excellent reviews of these historical conduit studies and can be reviewed for further detail.

Summary

The literature is only beginning to elucidate the best indications for PNA compared with nerve conduits. Based on the current available data, the use of nerve conduits for nerve gaps of less than 10 mm can provide meaningful sensory recovery.[22,26,27,37] The use of PNA for providing meaningful sensory recovery is supported by the current body of literature for digital nerve gaps of 10 mm or more.[22,31–35] The maximal nerve gap at which no meaningful recovery can be attained has yet to be determined; however, with further studies produced from the RANGER registry this question may be answered.

REFERENCES

1. Baker M, Walsh SP2, Schwartz Z, et al. A review of polyvinyl alcohol and its uses in cartilage and orthopedic applications. J Biomed Mater Res B Appl Biomater 2012;100:1451–7.

2. Taleb C, Berner S, Mantovani Ruggiero G. First metacarpal resurfacing with polyvinyl alcohol implant in rhizarthrosis: Preliminary study. Chir Main 2014;33(3):189–95.

3. Ku DN, Braddon LG, Wootton DM. Poly(vinyl alcohol) cryogel. US Patent no. 5981826, 1999.

4. Swieszkowski W, Ku DN, Bersee HE, et al. An elastic material for cartilage replacement in an arthritic shoulder joint. Biomaterials 2006;27:1534–41.

5. Oka M, Ushio K, Kumar P, et al. Development of artificial articular cartilage. Proc Inst Mech Eng H 2000;214(1):59–68.

6. Murakami T, Higaki H, Sawae Y, et al. Adaptive multimode lubrication in natural synovial joints and artificial joints. Proc Inst Mech Eng H 1998; 212(1):23–35.

7. Miller MD, Thompson SR, Hart JA. Review of orthopedics 6th Edition, section 8: biomaterials and biomechanics. Philadelphia: Elsevier; 2012.

8. Safety and effectiveness of cartiva implant in the treatment of first CMC joint osteoarthritis (GRIP)". National Institutes of Health: US National Library of Medicine. Available at: Clinicaltrials.gov. Accessed July 14, 2018.

9. Safety and effectiveness of Cartiva implant in the treatment of first CMC joint osteoarthritis compared to LRTI (GRIP 2). Available at: https://clinicaltrials.gov/ct2/show/NCT03247439. Accessed July 14, 2018.

10. Daniels TR, Younger AS, Penner MJ, et al. Midterm outcomes of polyvinyl alcohol hydrogel hemiarthroplasty of the first metatarsophalangeal joint in advanced hallux rigidus. Foot Ankle Int 2017;38(3):243–7.

11. Baumhauer JF, Singh D, Glazebrook M, et al, CARTIVA Motion Study Group. Prospective, randomized, multi-centered clinical trial assessing safety and efficacy of a synthetic cartilage implant versus first metatarsophalangeal arthrodesis in advanced hallux rigidus. Foot Ankle Int 2016;37:457–69.

12. Yan Y, Wood MD, Hunter DA, et al. The effect of short nerve grafts in series on axonal regeneration across isografts or acellular nerve allografts. J Hand Surg Am 2016;41(6):e113–21.

13. Hundepool CA, Nijhuis THJ, Kotsougiani D, et al. Optimizing decellularization techniques to create a new nerve allograft: an in vitro study using rodent nerve segments. Neurosurg Focus 2017;42(3):E4.

14. Ide C, Osawa T, Tohyama K. Nerve regeneration through allogeneic nerve grafts, with special reference to the role of the Schwann cell basal lamina. Prog Neurobiol 1990;34:1–38.

15. Graham JB, Xue QS, Neubauer D, et al. A chondroitinase-treated, decellularized nerve allograft compares favorably to the cellular isografts in rat peripheral nerve repair. J Neurodegener Regen 2009;2(1):19–29.

16. Hudson TW, Liu SY, Schmidt CE. Engineering an improved acellular nerve graft via optimized chemical processing. Tissue Eng 2004;10:1346–58.

17. Krekoski CA, Neubauer D, Zuo J, et al. Axonal regeneration into acellular nerve grafts is enhanced by degradation of chondroitin sulfate proteoglycan. J Neurosci 2001;21(6):6206–13.

18. Neubauer D, Graham JB, Muir D. Chondroitinase treatment increases the effective length of acellular nerve grafts. Exp Neurol 2007;207:163–70.

19. Sondell M, Lundborg G, Kanje M. Regeneration of the rat sciatic nerve into allografts made acellular through chemical extraction. Brain Res 1998;795: 44–54.

20. Whitlock EL, Tuffaha SH, Luciano JP, et al. Processed allograft and type I collagen conduits for repair of peripheral nerve gaps. Muscle Nerve 2009;787–99.

21. Pollins AC, Richard B, Boyer RB, et al. Comparing processed nerve allografts and assessing their capacity to retain and release nerve growth factor. Ann Plast Surg 2018;81:198–202.

22. Means KR, Rinker BD, Higgins JP, et al. A multicenter, prospective, randomized, pilot study of outcomes for digital nerve repair in the hand using hollow conduit compared with processed allograft nerve. Hand 2016;11(2):144–51.

23. Hoganson DM, Owens GE, O'Doherty EM, et al. Preserved extracellular matrix components and retained biological activity in decellularized porcine mesothelium. Biomaterials 2010;31:6934–40.

24. Meek MF, Coert JH. US Food and Drug Administration/Conformit Europe-approved absorbable nerve conduits for clinical repair of peripheral and cranial nerves. Ann Plast Surg 2008;60:110–6.

25. Nihsen ES, Johnson CE, Hiles MC. Bioactivity of small intestinal submucosa and oxidized regenerated cellulose/collagen. Adv Skin Wound Care 2008;21(10):479–86.

26. Rinker B, Liau JY. A prospective randomized study comparing woven polyglycolic acid and autogenous vein conduits for reconstruction of digital nerve gaps. J Hand Surg Am 2011;36(5):775–81.

27. Safa B, Buncke G. Autograft substitutes: conduits and processed nerve allografts. Hand Clin 2016;32:127–40.

28. Moore AM, Kasukurthi R, Magill CK, et al. Limitations of conduits in peripheral nerve repairs. Hand (N Y) 2009;4:180–6.

29. Chiriac S, Facca S, Diaconu M, et al. Experience of using the bioresorbable copolyester poly(DLlactide- epsilon-caprolactone) nerve conduit guide

Neurolac for nerve repair in peripheral nerve defects: report on a series of 28 lesions. J Hand Surg Eur Vol 2012;37:342–9.

30. Isaacs J. Treatment of acute peripheral nerve injuries: current concepts. J Hand Surg 2010;35A: 491–7.

31. Karabekmez FE, Duymaz A, Moran SL. Early clinical outcomes with the use of decellularized nerve allograft for repair of sensory defects within the hand. Hand (N Y) 2009;4:245–9.

32. Guo Y, Chen G, Tian G, et al. Sensory recovery following decellularized nerve allograft transplantation for digital nerve repair. J Plast Surg Hand Surg 2013;47:451–3.

33. Taras JS, Amin N, Patel N, et al. Allograft reconstruction for digital nerve loss. J Hand Surg Am 2013;38:1965–71.

34. Cho MS, Rinker BD, Weber RV, et al. Functional outcome following nerve repair in the upper extremity using processed nerve allograft. J Hand Surg Am 2012;37:2340–9.

35. Rinker BD, Zoldos J, Weber RV, et al. Use of processed nerve allograft to repair nerve injuries greater than 25 mm in the hand. Ann Plast Surg 2017;78:S292–5.

36. Weber RA, Breidenbach WC, Brown RE, et al. A randomized prospective study of polyglycolic acid conduits for digital nerve reconstruction in humans. Plast Reconstr Surg 2000;106:1036–45.

37. Taras JS, Jacoby SM, Lincoski CJ. Reconstruction of digital nerves with collagen conduits. J Hand Surg Am 2011;36(9):1441–6.

38. Lohmeyer JA, Kern Y, Schmauss D, et al. Prospective clinical study on digital nerve repair with collagen nerve conduits and review of literature. J Reconstr Microsurg 2014;30(4):227–34.

39. Schmauss D, Finck T, Liodaki E, et al. Is nerve regeneration after reconstruction with collagen nerve conduits terminated after 12 months? The long-term follow-up of two prospective clinical studies. J Reconstr Microsurg 2014;30:561–8.

Shoulder and Elbow

Safety and Efficacy of Intraoperative Computer-Navigated Versus Non-Navigated Shoulder Arthroplasty at a Tertiary Referral

Ian Barrett, MD*, Anna Ramakrishnan, MS,
Emilie Cheung, MD

KEYWORDS

- GPS navigation • Shoulder arthroplasty • Reverse shoulder arthroplasty
- Component placement • Computer navigation

KEY POINTS

- Optimal functioning and longevity of total and reverse shoulder arthroplasty are reliant on accurate and precise glenoid placement.
- Ideal and reproducible positioning of the glenoid component is difficult to achieve using standard instrumentation.
- Computer navigation technology enhances surgical planning and can aid surgeons in obtaining optimal glenoid positioning; this is especially true in cases of complex deformity.
- Using a positioning system does not significantly increase surgical time.

INTRODUCTION

The shoulder joint is unique in that it has the greatest range of motion of any joint in the body. To accomplish this feat, the shoulder relies on an intricate interplay between the soft tissue and bony structures. The bulk of inquiry into the biomechanics of the shoulder looks specifically at the reciprocal relationship of the rotator cuff and the deltoid. The deltoid muscle functions as the primary shoulder elevator in the scapular plane. Proper functioning of the muscle relies on maintaining appropriate tension and lever arm throughout the range of motion. No standard has yet been developed to determine the ideal native deltoid tension, but increased tension seen after placement of reverse shoulder arthroplasty can dramatically increase the efficiency of forward elevation. Changes in deltoid tension are typically inferred in the literature from changes in the distance from the acromion to the deltoid tuberosity or as a function of arm lengthening. Although exploiting deltoid efficiency is possible with increasing the muscle lever arm, there are significant disadvantages to overtensioning as well. Overstretched deltoids show progressive signs of denervation with successive electromyography observations, and increased tension on the origin of the muscle is associated with acromial fracture after arthroplasty.[1]

The rotator cuff works in tandem with the deltoid and provides concavity-compression force throughout range of motion, keeping the humeral head centered with respect to the glenoid. Rotator cuff deficiency results in superior migration of the humeral head in relation to

Disclosure Statement: The senior author E. Cheung is a consultant for Exactech (Gainesville, FL).
Department of Orthopedic Surgery, Stanford University, 450 Broadway Street, Redwood City, CA 94062, USA
* Corresponding author.
E-mail address: ianjsbarrett@gmail.com

the acromion. It is for this reason that rotator cuff–deficient shoulders demonstrate eccentric wear patterns, most characteristically increased superior glenoid wear and acetabularization of the acromion.[2] Recent studies in cadaveric models have demonstrated increased translation of the humerus up to 130% in rotator cuff–deficient shoulders.[3]

Standard total shoulder arthroplasty relies on maintaining the anatomic relationship between the rotator cuff and the deltoid. In the absence of the compressive forces stabilizing the humeral component on the glenoid tray, standard shoulder arthroplasties show overwhelmingly poor clinical outcomes and range of motion. Furthermore, rapid loosening and failure are expected because of the superior impingement and levering on the glenoid component.

In reverse total shoulder arthroplasty (RTSA), the fixed-fulcrum design of the reverse allows the compressive forces to be provided by the deltoid. The rotator cuff–deficient shoulder is able to function because the deltoid is able to function efficiently to provide overhead motion. Relative medialization of the center of rotation provided by the RTSA also reduces sheer forces across the glenoid baseplate to prevent early loosening.

Clinical outcomes following total shoulder arthroplasty rely on reconstruction of patient anatomy. Patients with improperly positioned implants are at a higher risk for limitations in range of motion, risk of dislocation, increased pain, and early loosening.[4,5] The component position also affects the risk of scapular notching in RTSA.[6] Most implants in malposition occur on the glenoid side; therefore, this has been the primary focus of efforts to improve methods of anatomic placement.

Defining the optimal position of the glenoid component has been a source of controversy since the inception of shoulder arthroplasty but has recently been brought into focus by several biomechanical and clinical studies. The current body of literature suggests that there are 3 aspects of glenoid positioning to consider when implanting glenoid-sided components for both reverse and total shoulder arthroplasty: containment, version, and inclination.

The principle of containment is intuitive and in line with general orthopedic principles of load sharing and bone conservation. Well-positioned implants should have congruent osseous backside support of greater than 90% of the implant surface and full bony containment of the peg or keel components with the least amount of reaming possible. This is the same for both total and reverse implants, although screw fixation of reverse components and altered sheer forces at the glenoid interface allow for more flexibility in situations where there is significant bone loss.

The anatomic version of the glenoid has been shown to vary between 1° and 9° of retroversion.[7] Long-term clinical studies demonstrate a greater incidence of loosening when the glenoid component is retroverted greater than 15°.[8] This loosening is thought to arise from a variety of factors. One concern is that shoulders with preoperative posterior subluxation will result in a high strain loading environment along the glenoid component contributing to failure. Another concern is that when there is eccentric reaming to correct for excessive retroversion, the subchondral plate is reamed away, leaving a soft cancellous bone surface on which the glenoid has insufficient support.

Consensus evidence indicates that an acceptable version is between 5° of anteversion and 15° of retroversion with most investigators aiming for between 0° and 10°.[9] Native inclination of the glenoid varies between 4° and 12°.[10] Inclination may affect range of motion after shoulder arthroplasty by increasing the arch of motion before humeral impingement on the acromion. Less than 20° of inclination is considered acceptable after total shoulder arthroplasty.[9]

Anatomic placement of the glenoid component with traditional methods has been shown to be very difficult even for experienced surgeons with modern instrumentation.[11] The overwhelming tendency is for surgeons to excessively revert components, likely as a result of failure to recognize the severity of the posterior wear present.[9] Although the addition of computed tomography (CT) scans and 3-dimensional (3D) imaging techniques has greatly improved surgeon awareness of this issue, it remains difficult to appreciate and compensate for intraoperatively.[12]

In a subset of cases, altered patient anatomy may limit glenoid exposure and prevent anatomic placement. Patients with prior trauma to the shoulder, including scapular neck fractures, proximal humerus malunions, or nonunions, may have a complex osseous deformity that makes using traditional bony and soft tissue landmarks difficult. Patients who previously underwent open or arthroscopic procedures on the shoulder may also have significantly altered tissue planes and excessive scar tissue, which limits exposure. The progression of glenoid deformity observed with severe osteoarthritis can also lead to complex osseous deformity and present similar problems during approach and implantation.

The Walch classification is the most commonly used system to identify common patterns of altered glenoid morphology preoperatively (**Fig. 1**). Although standard instrumentation is designed to adequately address the more common B1 and B2 morphology, the more recently defined B3 variant represents a unique challenge to the surgeon. The B3 glenoid represents the most severe form of pattern or erosion and is characterized by uni-concavity, absent paleoglenoid, medialization, retroversion, and subluxation of the humerus.[13] The preservation of concavity may conceal the increased subluxation potential and advanced bone loss associated with this variant. C-type glenoids, defined by greater than 25° of glenoid retroversion and absent posterior subluxation of the humerus, are thought to represent a normal variant or dysplastic feature and also represent a significant challenge to effectively placing components. In patients with a C-type glenoid, en face exposure of the glenoid is extremely difficult and the standard instrumentation that usually relies on a centralizing pin is difficult to implement.

Early navigation technology was shown to improve the accuracy of glenoid positioning but was plagued by bulky equipment and difficult implementation resulting in abandonment of the technology for several years. Current computer navigation technology has advanced considerably since its advent in the 1980s and has spurred renewed interest in this area.

METHODS

Multiple orthopedic device manufacturers, including Tornier, Biomet, Zimmer, DePuy, and Exactech, have developed proprietary software to assist with preoperative planning in shoulder arthroplasty. All systems work similarly in that they require specially formatted CT imaging obtained preoperatively to generate a 3D model of the bony scapula. The glenoid component can then be virtually implanted onto this 3D rendering of patients' anatomy before making any incisions. Using this method it is very simple to visualize the version, inclination, and containment of the implant and determine whether augmented components are necessary (**Fig. 2**). Each system has slight variations in the instrumentation, user interface, and software capabilities but ultimately provides similar information to the treating surgeon.

Current best practice models established by expert consensus advocate for preoperative CT scanning regardless of whether navigation technology is used; thus, this does not incur increased radiation exposure or cost for patients.[14] Even without the use of patient-specific guides or instrument-guided navigation, the use of 3D software to virtually implant the glenoid component has been shown in multiple studies to improve the final position and reduce the incidence of component perforation.[12,14,15]

Only one commercially available system, GPS (Exactech, Gainesville, FL), allows for intraoperative navigation of the component position. Similar to technologies seen in hip and knee arthroplasty, the GPS system uses a fixed point on patients' anatomy combined with input from the surgeon to create a stereotactic map of patients. All instrumentation is then referenced to this 3D mapping and correlated with the preoperative plan to ensure precise placement in the intended location.

Intraoperatively there are several techniques that should be applied when using GPS technology to enhance the speed and ease of the procedure. The incision will begin approximately 1

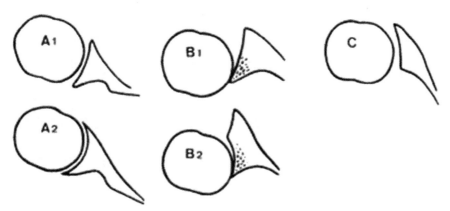

Fig. 1. Walch classification. (*From* Walch G, Badet R, Boulahia A, et al. Morphologic study of the glenoid in primary glenohumeral osteoarthritis. J Arthroplasty 1999;14(6):757; with permission.)

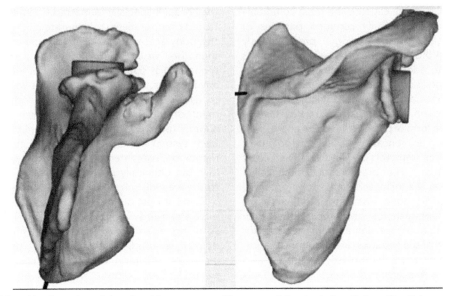

Fig. 2. Virtual implantation of the glenoid component. (*Courtesy of* Exactech, Inc, Gainesville, FL.)

to 2 cm proximal to the standard deltopectoral incision to allow access to the coracoid. Once adequately exposed, the coracoid should be isolated using Hohmann retractors and the cautery used to strip periosteum off the superior aspect; this will provide a landing zone for the tracker (Fig. 3).

Once the tracker is placed on the coracoid process, the next step is to reference the preoperative 3D scan against the exposed anatomy. This step is achieved by using a probe to identify standard bony landmarks as directed by the software (Fig. 4). This represents the greatest increase in time associated with the use of navigation technology. According to unpublished data, there was an increase in case time of approximately 6 minutes. Once the bony landmarks are registered, the standard instrumentation can be used in a navigated fashion to ensure

the optimal angle and depth of reaming according to the predefined plan (Fig. 5).

RESULTS

Long-term clinical studies comparing navigated and anatomic glenoid placement are still forthcoming, but early results are promising. Multiple studies have confirmed that simply using 3D technology platforms to virtually implant the glenoid preoperatively is helpful in improving surgeon accuracy.[12,14,15] This point is especially true in cases of severe glenoid deformity whereby standard 2-dimensional imaging is significantly less accurate.[16] Intraoperative guidance has been shown in cadaveric specimens to further improve the accuracy of placement. In a study looking at 16 cadaveric shoulders randomized to traditional or computer-assisted glenoid

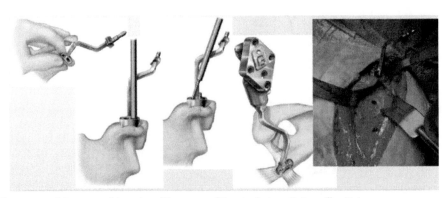

Fig. 3. Placement of the coracoid tracker. (*Courtesy of* Exactech, Inc, Gainesville, FL.)

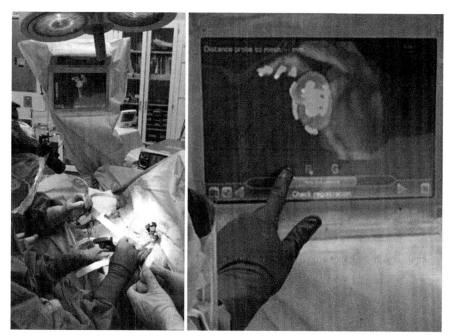

Fig. 4. Stereotactic mapping of glenoid face to 3D recon image.

implantation, the assisted group demonstrated significantly less version deviation. Most deviation seen in the traditional method could be attributed to errors in initial drilling.[11]

A comprehensive review of the literature examining intraoperative navigation confirmed superior accuracy in glenoid placement.[17]

Three-dimensional planning was also associated with greater use of augmented implants, most likely as a result of better understanding of patient anatomic retroversion.[14]

In vivo studies looking at the accuracy of glenoid placement confirm the superiority of guided techniques demonstrated in cadaveric

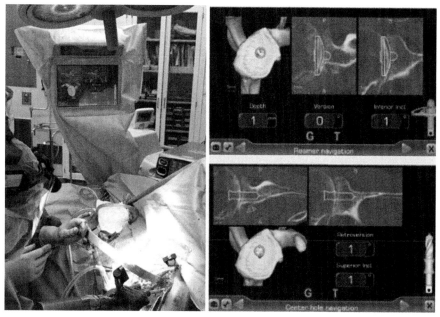

Fig. 5. Using 3D navigation to guide drilling of the central peg and reaming of the glenoid. Navigation provides feedback on implant positioning in all 3 radiographic planes as well as information about implant retroversion and tilt.

models. In a prospective trial looking at 31 patients randomized to either a conventional surgical technique combined with 3D planning software or patient-specific instrumentation, the investigators found that the PSI group had significantly decreased deviation from the templated plan. The investigators reported that the most advantageous use of PSI was in patients with retroversion greater than 16°.[18] The same results were seen when looking specifically at intraoperative guidance techniques. A study of 14 paired scapulohumeral cadaver specimens showed the range of error for version with guided techniques to be 8° versus 12° without. Neither group in this study had perforation of the central peg, but there were several screws in malposition in the control group.[19]

To date there is no published literature looking specifically at the difference between computer-navigated and traditional implantation. Cross-sectional data pending publication from the authors' institution (data not yet published) looked at surgical times in matched patient groups of that underwent shoulder arthroplasty with (n = 36) and without GPS navigation (n = 32) with an average follow-up of 6 months. In this group, GPS-navigated shoulders required 6 minutes or 9.5% additional surgical time on average (47–175 minutes total) (Fig. 6). The use of augmented components was equal between the two groups (2 patients in each group) requiring posterior augmentation. Intraoperative navigation had to be abandoned because of failure of the instrumentation to function in 1 out of 36 patients (2.7%) in the GPS arm. The difference in length of stay following surgery was not significant between the two groups. There were 2 incidents of intraoperative coracoid fracture (5.5%) reported in the GPS group.

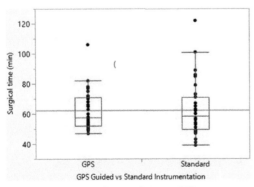

Fig. 6. Comparison of surgical times. GPS versus standard instrumentation.

DISCUSSION

Although the long-term clinical benefits of navigated shoulder arthroplasty have yet to be seen, there are several benefits that are already apparent. For one, the accuracy of glenoid placement is superior to traditional methods even in the hands of expert surgeons. This accuracy will allow surgeons who do not have the depth of experience to accurately and confidently position the glenoid. Nearly 50% of total shoulder arthroplasties in the country are performed at centers where less than 5 of these operations are performed yearly. This point may represent a significant advantage to average arthroplasty patients.[20] Low-volume institutions would also benefit significantly from the ability to anticipate the need for augmented implants, as these would typically need to be ordered in advance of the case.

Presumably the more accurate placement of the glenoid will allow for enhanced long-term survivorship of the implant and decrease complication rates. For example, screw malposition in RTSA is a common complication and can carry with it some significant risks. At minimum, it may damage the suprascapular nerve or cause a stress riser at the base of the scapular spine, which makes the scapular susceptible to fracture. At its worse, aberrant screw penetration can cause major neurovascular injury.[21]

Based on basic science studies, navigated technology would also decrease the complications seen in anatomic total shoulder arthroplasty. The most obvious is avoiding malposition of the glenoid component and the attendant problems with loosening or restriction in shoulder range of motion.

Finally, navigation technology represents an important teaching tool for trainees. The interactive software allows learners to understand the 3D shape of the scapula in real time and receive instantaneous feedback about the position of the component and their screws. The technology also benefits teachers in that they can feel comfortable allowing trainees to practice their skills while still maintaining a clear understanding of the operative field and giving them the ability to intercede if early.

The drawbacks of navigated technology include increased cost and increased intraoperative time. The increased cost is manifested in a significant upfront investment in the navigation technology but is also potentially bolstered by increased usage of more expensive augmented components. The time cost of navigated technology is significant upfront but does decrease over time largely because of increased surgeon experience. Finally, there is a small but significant risk of coracoid fracture due to tracker placement: 5.5% in this series. Of the 2 patients who sustained a fracture in the study group, each was noted to have subtle thinning of the coracoid and low bone density on postoperative review of the radiographs. Based on this observation, it is recommended that surgeons take particular care to identify patients with at-risk coracoid morphology before indicating the use of navigation.

The future of navigation technology in shoulder arthroplasty lies in the validation of improved clinical outcomes versus traditional methods. Larger-scale prospective randomized trials would clarify the importance of navigation technology in extending the longevity and function of the arthroplasty.

REFERENCES

1. Lädermann A, Walch G, Lubbeke A, et al. Influence of arm lengthening in reverse shoulder arthroplasty. J Shoulder Elbow Surg 2012;21:336–41.
2. Walker M, Brooks J, Willis M, et al. How reverse shoulder arthroplasty works. Clin Orthop Relat Res 2011;469:2440–51.
3. Kawano Y, Matsumura N, Murai A, et al. Evaluation of the translation distance of the glenohumeral joint and the function of the rotator cuff on its translation: a cadaveric study. Arthroscopy 2018;34(6):1776–84.
4. Flurin P-H, Roche CP, Wright TW, et al. Correlation between clinical outcomes and anatomic reconstruction with anatomic total shoulder arthroplasty. Bull Hosp Jt Dis 2015;73(Suppl 1):S92–8.
5. Shapiro TA, McGarry MH, Gupta R, et al. Biomechanical effects of glenoid retroversion in total shoulder arthroplasty. J Shoulder Elbow Surg 2007;16:90–5.
6. Simovitch RW. Predictors of scapular notching in patients managed with the delta III reverse total shoulder replacement. J Bone Joint Surg Am 2007;89:588.
7. Matsumura N, Ogawa K, Kobayashi S, et al. Morphologic features of humeral head and glenoid version in the normal glenohumeral joint. J Shoulder Elbow Surg 2014;23:1724–30.
8. Ho JC, Sabesan VJ, Iannotti JP. Glenoid component retroversion is associated with osteolysis. J Bone Joint Surg Am 2013;95:e82.
9. Gregory TM, Sankey A, Augereau B, et al. Accuracy of glenoid component placement in total shoulder arthroplasty and its effect on clinical and radiological outcome in a retrospective, longitudinal, monocentric open study. PLoS One 2013;8:2–8.
10. Churchill RS, Brems JJ, Kotschi H. Glenoid size, inclination, and version: an anatomic study. J Shoulder Elbow Surg 2001;10:327–32.
11. Nguyen D, Ferreira LM, Brownhill JR, et al. Improved accuracy of computer assisted glenoid implantation in total shoulder arthroplasty: an in-vitro randomized controlled trial. J Shoulder Elbow Surg 2009;18:907–14.
12. Berhouet J, Gulotta LV, Dines DM, et al. Preoperative planning for accurate glenoid component positioning in reverse shoulder arthroplasty. Orthop Traumatol Surg Res 2017;103:407–13.
13. Chan K, Knowles NK, Chaoui J, et al. Characterization of the Walch B3 glenoid in primary osteoarthritis. J Shoulder Elbow Surg 2017;26:909–14.
14. Werner BS, Hudek R, Burkhart KJ, et al. The influence of three-dimensional planning on decision-making in total shoulder arthroplasty. J Shoulder Elbow Surg 2017;26:1477–83.
15. Iannotti JP, Weiner S, Rodriguez E, et al. Three-dimensional imaging and templating improve glenoid implant positioning. J Bone Joint Surg Am 2015;97:651–8.
16. Iannotti JP, Greeson C, Downing D, et al. Effect of glenoid deformity on glenoid component placement in primary shoulder arthroplasty. J Shoulder Elbow Surg 2012;21:48–55.
17. Sadoghi P, Vavken J, Leithner A, et al. Benefit of intraoperative navigation on glenoid component positioning during total shoulder arthroplasty. Arch Orthop Trauma Surg 2015;135:41–7.
18. Hendel MD, Bryan JA, Barsoum WK, et al. Comparison of patient-specific instruments with standard surgical instruments in determining glenoid component position: a randomized prospective clinical trial. J Bone Joint Surg Am 2012;94:2167–75.
19. Verborgt O, De Smedt T, Vanhees M, et al. Accuracy of placement of the glenoid component in reversed shoulder arthroplasty with and without navigation. J Shoulder Elbow Surg 2011;20:21–6.
20. Schairer WW, Nwachukwu BU, Lyman S, et al. National utilization of reverse total shoulder arthroplasty in the United States. J Shoulder Elbow Surg 2015;24:91–7.
21. Molony DC, Cassar Gheiti AJ, Kennedy J, et al. A cadaveric model for suprascapular nerve injury during glenoid component screw insertion in reverse-geometry shoulder arthroplasty. J Shoulder Elbow Surg 2011;20:1323–7.

Technologies to Augment Rotator Cuff Repair

Anand M. Murthi, MD*, Manesha Lankachandra, MD

KEYWORDS

- Rotator cuff repair • Platelet-rich plasma • Allograft scaffold • Synthetic scaffold • Stem cells

KEY POINTS

- The consensus of the current literature seems to be that platelet-rich plasma (PRP) may provide some clinical benefit in rotator cuff repair, but there remains high variability among different PRP products and preparations.
- Like PRP, the efficacy of the bone marrow aspirate concentration preparation depends on the expression of various cytokines and signaling molecules and the product used.
- Various scaffolds and grafts, both biological and synthetic, are available to provide structural support for the repair. Their effects and results vary depending on graft type.

Retear rates after rotator cuff repair vary widely, depending on the tear type and size as well as patient factors, such as age and health comorbidities. Earlier research has shown that pain relief and satisfaction can reliably be achieved despite tendon healing.[1–3] A 2014 meta-analysis of level I and II data showed some significant difference in some outcome measures, but these differences did not reach clinical importance. Importantly, the influence of age and occupation were not evaluated, and most of the studied tears were small. Patients with intact repairs were also found to have greater strength than those with retears.[4] The goal of surgical rotator cuff repair remains a tension-free repair that can withstand the functional demands of patients during the postoperative healing and rehabilitative phase. Tendon to bone healing is notoriously fickle, and the fibrous scar tissue that creates this repair lacks the mechanical strength and elasticity of native tendon.[5,6] New technologies seek to improve tendon to bone healing with the addition of platelet-rich plasma (PRP), stem cells, and biological and synthetic grafts (Figs. 1 and 2).

After physical reattachment of rotator cuff tendons to their insertion sites, the cells and biological factors involved in healing the repaired bone to tendon interface derive from surrounding connective tissues.

PRP is an autologous blood product with platelet concentrations greater than the baseline values.[7] It is created through plasmapheresis whereby platelets and plasma are separated from white blood cells (WBCs) and red blood cells. Commercial preparation methods vary, with varying amounts of platelets and WBCs in the final product. Moreover, most users do not perform cell counts on the whole blood or PRP products to evaluate these differences clinically.

The optimal ratio of PRP products has not been established, but a recent basic science study does suggest that leukocyte-poor PRP promotes more normal collagen matrix synthesis and decreases more potentially harmful cytokines and inflammatory markers than high-leukocyte PRP preparations.[8]

In the perioperative setting, PRP is used to stimulate healing at the tendon-bone interface. In a meta-analysis of 5 studies, Chahal and

The authors declare no potential conflict of interest related to this article.

Department of Orthopaedics, MedStar Union Memorial Hospital, 3333 North Calvert Street, Suite 400, Baltimore, MD 21218, USA

* Corresponding author. Department of Orthopaedics, MedStar Union Memorial Hospital, 3333 North Calvert Street, Suite 400, Baltimore, MD 21218.

E-mail address: amurthi14@hotmail.com

Orthop Clin N Am 50 (2019) 103–108

https://doi.org/10.1016/j.ocl.2018.08.005

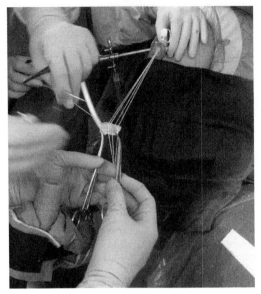

Fig. 1. A synthetic graft outside of the body, ready to be passed into the subacromial space through a lateral portal.

colleagues[9] showed patient-reported outcomes were no different between the two groups and the risk of retear was not significantly changed. A larger meta-analysis of 11 studies also similarly showed no difference in retear rates and patient outcomes in patients treated with PRP and controls.[10] There was, however, a statistically significant reduction in retear rates with larger tears (greater than 3 cm) that were treated with double-row repair and PRP. A 2018 meta-analysis of PRP and platelet-rich fibrin by Hurley and colleagues[11] showed that the use of PRP improved tendon healing rates in tears of all sizes. The increase in the number of studies available for review regarding the use of PRP products over recent years allowed the

investigators to subgroup PRP and platelet-rich fibrin; they found that although the use of PRP resulted in improved healing rates and functional outcomes, the use of platelet-rich fibrin had no beneficial effect on tendon healing or outcomes.

A 2012 study of 37 patients also evaluated the effects of platelet-rich fibrin on repair integrity following rotator cuff repairs at high risk of failure (older patients, larger tears, and higher Goutallier scores). Retear rates were higher in the study group versus the control group. Functional outcome scores were similar in the two groups.[12]

The consensus of current literature seems to be that PRP in rotator cuff repair does provide some clinical benefit, improving healing rates in tears of various sizes and with variable patient factors. That this consensus has changed considerably over the past decade shows the evolving nature of both PRP products and how they are being used by surgeons. There are still no clear guideline regarding the characterization of PRP products, both in clinical use and scientific reporting. That some PRP-related products (platelet-rich fibrin, for example) are clearly not beneficial also underscores the heterogeneity of PRP preparations and the difficulty in making generalizations regarding the use of PRP in rotator cuff repair.

Similar to PRP, the use of stem cell preparations at the bone-tendon repair interface also seeks to create a favorable milieu of chemical signaling. Snyder and Burns'[13] crimson duvet is a well-known technique to create a collection of stem cells and cytokines at the repair site, using similar principles as microfracture. Basic science research in a rat model showed increased mesenchymal stem cells in the drilling group versus the control group, and the ultimate force

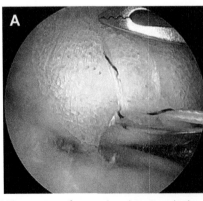
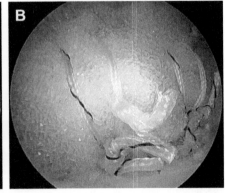

Fig. 2. (A) The same graft now placed against the bursal side of the rotator cuff repair. (B) It is tied down against the tendon bone interface.

to failure was significantly higher in the drilling group at 4 and 8 weeks.[14] A similar study in rabbits also showed increased force to failure at 8 and 16 weeks, and histologic analysis showed thicker collagen bundles and more fibrocartilage in the microfracture group.[15]

In humans studies, clinical outcomes have been similar in patients undergoing microfracture or other marrow-stimulating techniques.[16–18] Milano and colleagues[17] reported on 80 patients, 40 who were randomized to receive microfracture with rotator cuff repair and 40 patients who underwent cuff repair alone. At a mean follow-up of roughly 2 years, Constant scores were similar in the two groups. There was no difference in healing rates between the two groups, though subgroup analysis did show better healing rates for large tears in the microfracture group. Taniguchi and colleagues[18] also showed improved repair integrity in large and massive cuff tears using bone marrow stimulation, despite similar results between groups in small and medium tears.

Mesenchymal stem cells from bone marrow can also be collected and concentrated from bone marrow and injected back at the site of repair (Fig. 3). Like PRP, there are multiple systems from multiple companies. Like PRP, the efficacy of the bone marrow aspirate concentration preparation depends on the expression of various cytokines and signaling molecules.

The site of harvest of these bone marrow cells also varies. Bone marrow aspirate is commonly harvested from the greater tuberosity (Fig. 4), which minimizes donor site morbidity and increases surgical time. However, Hernigou and colleagues[19] showed that bone marrow aspirate from this site might have fewer mesenchymal

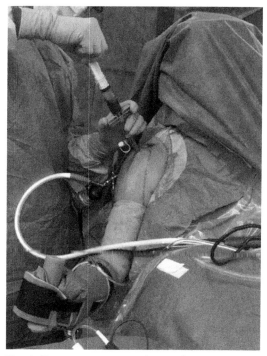

Fig. 4. Bone marrow aspirate harvest from the greater tuberosity. A Jamshidi needle is used through a lateral portal; no other incisions are necessary.

stem cells in the setting of chronic rotator cuff tear.

Although mesenchymal stem cells from bone marrow concentrate can differentiate into tendon cells, the clinical significance of this finding in rotator cuff surgery is unclear. Animal studies have shown that the bone marrow-derived cells were active at the site of repair, but results regarding improvement in the mechanical strength of the repair are mixed.[20–22] In humans, 2 recent studies show decreased retear rates in both primary and revision settings using bone marrow aspirate.[19,23]

In addition to maximizing the biological components of the repair, various scaffold and grafts, both biological and synthetic, are available to provide structural support for the repair. This support becomes especially important when patient factors result in poor-quality tissue at the site of repair. Neviaser and colleagues[24] initially described the use of graft material in rotator cuff repair in the 1970s to bridge in irreparable repair. This idea has recently been taken further with the idea of superior capsular reconstruction; but graft material is more commonly used to reinforce a repair with poor quality tissue, rather than to bridge a gap between tendon and bone. The use of grafts as scaffolds can

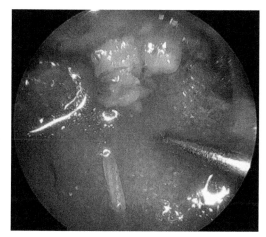

Fig. 3. Bone marrow aspirate concentrate injected into and around the synthetic graft and repair.

generally be split into products that use biological material, usually human or animal extracellular matrix, and those that use synthetic materials.

In vitro research has shown that the structural makeup and mechanical properties of both biological and synthetic grafts is relatively dissimilar from native rotator cuff tendon. Smith and colleagues[25] evaluated 7 scaffolds, comparing their mechanical properties with a cadaver supraspinatus tendon. Synthetic grafts fared better in load to failure tests when compared with biological grafts, but neither matched native supraspinatus tendon. The investigators suggested that one reason for this dissimilarity may lie in the origin of these grafts for uses outside of the shoulder, and further research into grafts designed to mimic the rotator cuff tendons may hold promise.

Histologic studies show evidence of increased cell adhesion and proliferation, depending on the graft type.[26] Arnoczky and colleagues[27] recently performed a retrospective study of 7 patients who underwent rotator cuff procedures with a bovine collagen graft and then underwent a repeat surgery with biopsy. At 5 weeks, biopsies showed host fibroblasts within the collagen implant. At 8 weeks, there was further host incorporation within the implant with linear organization of the host collagen fibers. At 3 months, biopsies showed further host incorporation of the implant as well as implant degradation. At 6 months, the remnants of the implant were gone and the tissue samples had the organized appearance of tendon, densely organized with parallel bundles of collagen fibers. In this study, at no point was there inflammatory or foreign body reaction within the sampled tissue.

The is a paucity of human studies on host response to synthetic scaffolds, but a canine study showed improved biomechanical function at 12 weeks. In this study, 8 dogs underwent bilateral shoulder surgery, with one side repaired and the other repaired and augmented with a polymer scaffold. At time zero, repair with augmentation increased load to failure; at 12 weeks, there was less tendon retraction and greater cross-sectional area. Histologic samples at 12 weeks also showed fibrous tissue ingrowth with an overall compatible host response.[28] A similar study in rats using a polycarbonate polyurethane patch showed no inflammatory response at 6 weeks as well as significant host tissue ingrowth.[29] Regarding the initial repair strength using a synthetic scaffold, a small cadaver study showed the ultimate load to failure was improved by 25% for rotator cuff repairs

augmented with a polyhydroxyalkanoate mesh. There was no difference in gap formation after cyclic loading.

Human studies show generally favorable outcomes with the use of biological grafts. In one of the few randomized controlled trials, Barber and colleagues[30] showed American Shoulder and Elbow Surgeons (ASES) and Constant scores were improved and cuff integrity was better maintained in patients who underwent repair plus augmentation with dermal allograft of their large (2 tendons) rotator cuff tears versus those who underwent repair alone. Intact repairs were found in 85% of the augmentation group versus 40% of the control group at a mean of 14 months postoperatively. The investigators also note that operative time was generally increased by 30 to 60 minutes in the augmentation group.

Other retrospective studies using biological grafts for bridging augmentation, especially in the setting of massive rotator cuff tears, also show good results. In a study of 45 patients with massive rotator cuff tears treated arthroscopically with a regenerative tissue matrix allograft augmentation using a bridging construct, Wong and colleagues[31] show improved University of California, Los Angeles and ASES scores as well as improved functionality at 2 years postoperatively. The average postoperative ASES score in this group was 84.1, and it is important to note that the technique used in this report involved bridging deficient rotator cuff tendons rather than augmenting tendon to bone repair. In a study of 24 patients with massive rotator cuff tears treated using a mini open technique with regenerative tissue matrix allograft, Gupta and colleagues[32] showed improved the Short Form 12 (SF-12) and ASES scores at 3 years postoperatively. The mean ASES scores improved from 66.6 to 88.7, and the mean SF-12 scores improved from 48.4 to 56.8. Neither of these reports had control groups, and it is important to note that the surgical technique used involved bridging a bone to tendon gap versus purely an augmentation of a tenuous repair.

In a revision setting, Petri and colleagues[33] showed significant improvement in the functional portion of the ASES after open, revision, biological patch augmentation. Patient satisfaction in this series was also high, with no patients requiring further surgery. In a larger review of 24 patients undergoing revision open rotator cuff repair with dermal allograft augmentation, 10 patients had MRI evidence of a retear at 50 months.[34] Based on ASES and simple assessment numeric evaluation (SANE) scores, excellent results were achieved in 24% of patients, good in 13%, fair in 21%, and poor in 42%. Interestingly, this study compared these outcomes with historical control of revision surgery without augmentation and found no significant improvements.

For synthetic scaffolds, one of the only studies with a control group compared open rotator cuff repair, repair with a collagen scaffold, and repair with a synthetic scaffold. The polypropylene patch augmentation of rotator cuff repair demonstrated significant improvement in the 36-month outcome in terms of function, strength, and retear rate.[35] Other case series as well have shown decreased pain, increased range of motion, and improvement in patient-reported outcomes.[36–38] Even in revision settings, case series have shown good results with synthetic grafts. Although retear rates in this population remain high, shoulder outcome scores significantly improved.[39]

Recent technology may allow improved healing rates in both simple and complex rotator cuff repair surgery. Understanding the nuances of biologics and grafting can allow surgeons to choose the appropriate augmentation techniques and products in their primary and revision rotator cuff repair patients. Many of these newer technologies still need to be studied in a prospective fashion to allow for a thorough understanding of their role in improved outcomes while factoring in the potential for added cost and risks.

REFERENCES

1. Boileau P, Brassart N, Watkinson DJ, et al. Arthroscopic repair of full-thickness tears of the supraspinatus: does the tendon really heal? J Bone Joint Surg Am 2005;87:1229–40.

2. Burkhart SS, Barth JR, Richards DP, et al. Arthroscopic repair of massive rotator cuff tears with stage 3 and 4 fatty degeneration. Arthroscopy 2007;23:347–54.

3. Jost B, Pfirrmann CW, Gerber C, et al. Clinical outcome after structural failure of rotator cuff repairs. J Bone Joint Surg Am 2000;82:304–14.

4. Russell RD, Knight JR, Mulligan E, et al. Structural integrity after rotator cuff repair does not correlate with patient function and pain: a meta-analysis. J Bone Joint Surg Am 2014;96:265–71.

5. Bunker DL, Ilie V, Ilie V, et al. Tendon to bone healing and its implications for surgery. Muscles Ligaments Tendons J 2014;4:343–50.

6. Rodeo SA. Biologic augmentation of rotator cuff tendon repair. J Shoulder Elbow Surg 2007;16: S191–7.

7. Hsu WK, Mishra A, Rodeo SR, et al. Platelet-rich plasma in orthopaedic applications: evidence-based recommendations for treatment. J Am Acad Orthop Surg 2013;21:739–48.

8. Cross JA, Cole BJ, Spatny KP, et al. Leukocyte-reduced platelet-rich plasma normalizes matrix metabolism in torn human rotator cuff tendons. Am J Sports Med 2015;43:2898–906.

9. Chahal J, Van Thiel GS, Mall N, et al. The role of platelet-rich plasma in arthroscopic rotator cuff repair: a systematic review with quantitative synthesis. Arthroscopy 2012;28:1718–27.

10. Warth RJ, Dornan GJ, James EW, et al. Clinical and structural outcomes after arthroscopic repair of full-thickness rotator cuff tears with and without platelet-rich product supplementation: a meta-analysis and meta-regression. Arthroscopy 2015; 31:306–20.

11. Hurley ET, Lim FD, Moran CJ, et al. The efficacy of platelet-rich plasma and platelet-rich fibrin in arthroscopic rotator cuff repair: a meta-analysis of randomized controlled trials. Am J Sports Med 2018. 363546517751397. [Epub ahead of print].

12. Bergeson AG, Tashjian RZ, Greis PE, et al. Effects of platelet-rich fibrin matrix on repair integrity of at-risk rotator cuff tears. Am J Sports Med 2012;40: 286–93.

13. Snyder S, Burns J. Rotator cuff healing and the bone marrow "crimson duvet." From clinical observations to science. Tech Shoulder Elbow Surg 2009; 10:130–7.

14. Kida Y, Morihara T, Matsuda K, et al. Bone marrow-derived cells from the footprint infiltrate into the repaired rotator cuff. J Shoulder Elbow Surg 2013; 22:197–205.

15. Bilsel K, Yildiz F, Kapicioglu M, et al. Efficacy of bone marrow-stimulating technique in rotator cuff repair. J Shoulder Elbow Surg 2017;26: 1360–6.

16. Jo CH, Shin JS, Park IW, et al. Multiple channeling improves the structural integrity of rotator cuff repair. Am J Sports Med 2013;41:2650–7.

17. Milano G, Saccomanno MF, Careri S, et al. Efficacy of marrow-stimulating technique in arthroscopic rotator cuff repair: a prospective randomized study. Arthroscopy 2013;29:802–10.

18. Taniguchi N, Suenaga N, Oizumi N, et al. Bone marrow stimulation at the footprint of arthroscopic surface-holding repair advances cuff repair integrity. J Shoulder Elbow Surg 2015;24:860–6.

19. Hernigou P, Merouse G, Duffiet P, et al. Reduced levels of mesenchymal stem cells at the tendon-bone interface tuberosity in patients with symptomatic rotator cuff tear. Int Orthop 2015;39: 1219–25.

20. Gulotta LV, Kovacevic D, Ehteshami JR, et al. Application of bone marrow-derived mesenchymal stem

cells in a rotator cuff repair model. Am J Sports Med 2009;37:2126–33.

21. Liu XN, Yang CJ, Kim JE, et al. Enhanced tendon-to-bone healing of chronic rotator cuff tears by bone marrow aspirate concentrate in a rabbit model. Clin Orthop Surg 2018;10:99–110.

22. Safi E, Ficklscherer A, Bondarava M, et al. Migration of mesenchymal stem cells of bursal tissue after rotator cuff repair in rats. Joints 2018;6:4–9.

23. Depres-Tremblay G, Chevrier A, Snow M, et al. Rotator cuff repair: a review of surgical techniques, animal models, and new technologies under development. J Shoulder Elbow Surg 2016;25:2078–85.

24. Neviaser JS, Neviaser RJ, Neviaser TJ. The repair of chronic massive ruptures of the rotator cuff of the shoulder by use of a freeze-dried rotator cuff. J Bone Joint Surg Am 1978;60:681–4.

25. Smith RDJ, Zargar N, Brown CP, et al. Characterizing the macro and micro mechanical properties of scaffolds for rotator cuff repair. J Shoulder Elbow Surg 2017;26:2038–46.

26. Ricchetti ET, Aurora A, Iannotti JP, et al. Scaffold devices for rotator cuff repair. J Shoulder Elbow Surg 2012;21:251–65.

27. Arnoczky SP, Bishai SK, Schofield B, et al. Histologic evaluation of biopsy specimens obtained after rotator cuff repair augmented with a highly porous collagen implant. Arthroscopy 2017;33:278–83.

28. Derwin KA, Codsi MJ, Milks RA, et al. Rotator cuff repair augmentation in a canine model with use of a woven poly-L-lactide device. J Bone Joint Surg Am 2009;91:1159–71.

29. Cole BJ, Gomoll AH, Yanke A, et al. Biocompatibility of a polymer patch for rotator cuff repair. Knee Surg Sports Traumatol Arthrosc 2007;15:632–7.

30. Barber FA, Burns JP, Deutsch A, et al. A prospective, randomized evaluation of acellular human dermal matrix augmentation for arthroscopic rotator cuff repair. Arthroscopy 2012;28:8–15.

31. Wong I, Burns J, Snyder S. Arthroscopic GraftJacket repair of rotator cuff tears. J Shoulder Elbow Surg 2010;19:104–9.

32. Gupta AK, Hug K, Berkoff DJ, et al. Dermal tissue allograft for the repair of massive irreparable rotator cuff tears. Am J Sports Med 2012;40:141–7.

33. Petri M, Warth RJ, Horan MP, et al. Outcomes after open revision repair of massive rotator cuff tears with biologic patch augmentation. Arthroscopy 2016;32:1752–60.

34. Sears BW, Choo A, Yu A, et al. Clinical outcomes in patients undergoing revision rotator cuff repair with extracellular matrix augmentation. Orthopedics 2015;38:e292–6.

35. Ciampi P, Scotti C, Nonis A, et al. The benefit of synthetic versus biological patch augmentation in the repair of posterosuperior massive rotator cuff tears: a 3-year follow-up study. Am J Sports Med 2014;42:1169–75.

36. Encalada-Diaz I, Cole BJ, Macgillivray JD, et al. Rotator cuff repair augmentation using a novel polycarbonate polyurethane patch: preliminary results at 12 months' follow-up. J Shoulder Elbow Surg 2011;20:788–94.

37. Nada AN, Debnath UK, Robinson DA, et al. Treatment of massive rotator-cuff tears with a polyester ligament (Dacron) augmentation: clinical outcome. J Bone Joint Surg Br 2010;92:1397–402.

38. Proctor CS. Long-term successful arthroscopic repair of large and massive rotator cuff tears with a functional and degradable reinforcement device. J Shoulder Elbow Surg 2014;23:1508–13.

39. Lenart BA, Martens KA, Kearns KA, et al. Treatment of massive and recurrent rotator cuff tears augmented with a poly-l-lactide graft, a preliminary study. J Shoulder Elbow Surg 2015;24:915–21.

Foot and Ankle

New Technology in the Treatment of Hallux Rigidus with a Synthetic Cartilage Implant Hemiarthroplasty

Judith F. Baumhauer, MD, MPH[a],*,
Timothy Daniels, MD, FRCSC[b],
Mark Glazebrook, MD, PHD, FRCSC[c]

KEYWORDS

- Synthetic cartilage implant • Hemiarthroplasty • Hallux rigidus • Great toe arthritis
- Hallux limitus • Interposition arthroplasty

KEY POINTS

- A 90% success rate equivalent to first metatarsophalangeal (MTP) fusion for pain relief and function can be achieved while maintaining great toe motion at 2 and 5 years.
- Surgeons should aim for 1.5 to 3 mm of implant observed outside the bone. Do not "bottom out" the step reamer.
- Good bone is important to maintain the implant position. Osteoporosis, large cysts, or structural lesions in the metatarsal head are contraindications to this procedure.
- Despite postoperative recovery being simpler with the implant than a first MTP fusion, the pain and functional improvement may require a minimum of 3 months to begin to improve with continued improvement over the following 6 to 12 months.
- If the patient has continued pain limiting function at 1 year after implant surgery, a revision surgery with simple implant removal and conversion to a fusion can be performed with the same pain relief and function as if the fusion had been done primarily.

INTRODUCTION

Great toe arthritis, called hallux rigidus or hallux limitus, is an extremely common condition leading to pain and activity limitations.[1,2] It has been estimated that nearly 80% of patients over the age of 50 will have some degree of great toe arthritis.[3] Women are more commonly affected than men, and 50% of the cases can be bilateral.[4,5] Up until 2016, the options for great toe arthritis included cheilectomy, capsular or commercial interposition arthroplasty with or without modified Keller resection arthroplasty, partial or total toe joint replacement, or first metatarsophalangeal (MTP) arthrodesis.[2,6,7] Because of the continued dissatisfaction and lack of consistently good results with these joint-sparing operations, the first MTP arthrodesis was considered the gold standard of treatment. Despite the arthrodesis providing excellent pain relief, the sacrifice of motion of the first MTP joint for activities as well as shoe

Disclosure Statement: The authors are Consultants for Cartiva; Cartiva Development Team.
[a] Ortho Department, University of Rochester School of Medicine and Dentistry, University of Rochester Medical Center, 601 Elmwood Avenue, Rochester, NY 14642, USA; [b] Division of Orthopaedic Surgery, St. Michael's Hospital, University of Toronto, 800-55 Queen Street East, Toronto, Ontario M5C 1R6, Canada; [c] Dalhousie University, Queen Elizabeth II Health Sciences Center, Halifax Infirmary, Room 4867, 1796 Summer Street, Halifax, Nova Scotia B3H 3A7, Canada
* Corresponding author.
E-mail address: JUDY_BAUMHAUER@URMC.ROCHESTER.EDU

wear choices drove foot and ankle surgeons to look for an alternative option. The alternative option needed to have several pivotal qualities, as follows:

1. The alternative option should maintain or improve great toe motion.
2. The alternative option should reduce pain similar to that seen with a first MTP arthrodesis.
3. The alternative option should provide patients the opportunity to return to functional activities such as sports and specifically running and jumping.
4. The alternative option should minimize bone resection so that conversion to a fusion would be possible and result in equivalent results as if a fusion had been done primarily.
5. The surgery should be simple and easily reproduced regardless of surgical experience.
6. If an implant is used, it needs to be durable, inert, and similar to the mechanical properties of cartilage to be friendly to the bone.

Based on these criteria, a hydrogel made up of polyvinyl alcohol and saline was identified from a clinical series of patients treated in Europe.[8] The implant size was 8 or 10 mm, and it was implanted into the metatarsal head and left approximately 1.5 mm proud to allow for distraction of the joint. The dorsal first metatarsal osteophytes and corresponding osteophytes at the base of the proximal phalanx were also resected. With the implant being smaller than the metatarsal head, there was a significant rim of cortical bone maintaining length of the metatarsal. In addition, the properties of the synthetic cartilage implant were very similar to cartilage and found to be significantly durable with cyclic loading and wear testing. Comprehensive histology testing as well as biomechanical testing coupled with the positive clinical series provided enough support to encourage 12 clinical sites in the United Kingdom and Canada to participate in a prospective randomized clinical trial comparing outcomes between the hydrogel implant to a first MTP arthrodesis in patients with advanced arthritis. The 2- and 5-year follow-up studies demonstrated equivalent pain relief and functional outcomes between the 2 treatments.[9,10]

INDICATIONS AND CONTRAINDICATIONS

The Cartiva Synthetic Cartilage Implant (Cartiva, Inc, Alpharetta, GA, USA) is intended for use in the treatment of patients with painful degenerative or posttraumatic arthritis (hallux rigidus or limitus) of the first MTP joint with or without the presence of mild hallux valgus. Synthetic cartilage implant hemiarthroplasty is not indicated in patients with painful sesamoid arthritis, active infection of the foot, known allergy to polyvinyl alcohol, weak bone or inadequate bone stock including patients with osteoporosis, osteopenia, or inflammatory arthroplasty. Patients who have had prior surgery such as a cheilectomy may have inadequate dorsal bone stock to contain a synthetic cartilage implant. Additional specific contraindications are listed in Box 1.

SETTING PATIENT EXPECTATIONS

Although the surgical procedure only has a few steps to insert the synthetic cartilage implant and there is no recommended immobilization of the foot after surgery beyond a postoperative shoe, the surgery does require the first MTP joint to be fully flexed to 90° to allow drilling of the bone, removal of the osteophytes and placement of the synthetic cartilage implant. With this degree of surgery, dissection, and motion preservation, it is known from the randomized clinical trial that patients will begin to experience pain improvement at 3 months, and this will continue for 1 year.[9] It is important to share with patients that this is the natural course of the recovery. It is the common belief of patients that "if I am back in my shoe I must have reached maximal medical improvement." This is not the case. As with any procedure, the more the

---

Box 1
Contraindications for synthetic cartilage implant hemiarthroplasty

Sesamoid arthritis

Active infection of the foot

Known allergy to polyvinyl alcohol

Inadequate bone stock of MTP joint

Osteoporosis or osteopenia

Avascular necrosis of MTP joint

Large osteochondral cyst at MTP joint

Active gout with tophi

Metabolic disorders leading to progressive deterioration of bone, including inflammatory arthropathies, Charcot arthropathy, uncontrolled diabetes

Tumors or foot deformities of the supporting bone structures

patient knows about what to expect after surgery, the easier the recovery progresses.

SURGICAL TECHNIQUE/PROCEDURE

Preoperative Planning

Preoperative planning should first begin with identifying patients who have failed common nonoperative treatment and meet the inclusion and exclusion criteria described above. Standing anteroposterior (A/P) and lateral radiographs should be taken and reviewed to assure proper indications and contraindications are met (Figs. 1A and 2A). The size of the metatarsal head should be measured in the axial and sagittal plane to allow estimation of the synthetic cartilage implant size (8 or 10 mm).

Preparation and Patient Positioning

General, regional, or local anesthesia can be used, and the patient should be placed in the supine position with a bump under the ipsilateral hip as needed to have the great toe facing up. The ankle and foot are prepared and draped in the usual sterile fashion.

Surgical Steps

Step 1

Surgical exposure of the MTP joint is accomplished using a dorsal surgical approach with an incision approximately 4 cm in length along the medial aspect of the extensor hallucis longus (EHL) tendon. The MTP arthrotomy is then made along the same line of the incision just medial to the EHL tendon, and dissection of the joint capsule is continued dorsally both medially and laterally to allow exposure of the MTP head (Fig. 3). At this point, an osteophyte resection of the proximal phalanx base and metatarsal (MT) head is performed leaving an intact MT cortical rim for size and stability to accept the 8- or 10-mm implant. Caution is advised to avoid excessive dorsal osteophyte resection of the cortical bone metatarsal head to avoid incomplete containment of the synthetic cartilage implant. A minimum of 2 mm of cortical circumferential bone is recommended to support the implant (Fig. 4).

Step 2

Center the concave end of the cannulated implant placer (8- or 10-mm size) on the

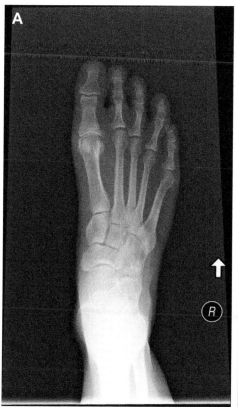
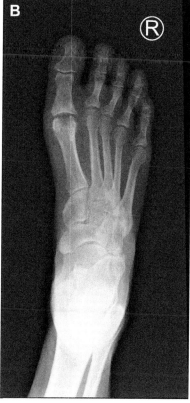

Fig. 1. (A) Preoperative standing A/P radiograph, and (B) postoperative A/P foot radiograph after Cartiva placement.

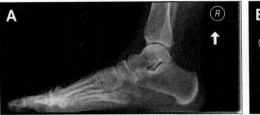
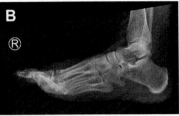

Fig. 2. (A) Preoperative standing lateral radiograph, and (B) postoperative lateral foot radiograph after Cartiva implant placement.

metatarsal head to allow placement of the guide pin in the central portion of the metatarsal head (**Fig. 5**). The position of this guide pin may be confirmed using intraoperative fluoroscopy imaging documenting central guide pin placement on the A/P and lateral images. Confirm there exists a minimum of 2 mm of cortical circumferential bone to support the implant and remove the cannulated implant placer leaving the guide pin in place in the metatarsal head.

An alternative asymmetric guide pin placement technique may be used to target synthetic cartilage implant placement at the maximum area of cartilage wear identifying the greatest point of load contact of the MT head. This asymmetric pin placement technique is accomplished using the concave end of the placer (8- or 10-mm size) positioned asymmetrically at the maximum cartilage wear area or the highest point of the MT head (**Fig. 6**). A minimum of 2 mm of cortical circumferential bone must be confirmed to exist to support the implant before removing the implant placer (**Fig. 7**).

Step 3

The MT head implantation site is created by advancing the appropriate sized step drill over the guide pin; start the drill before contacting the MT head. Ream the MT head until the step drill is approximately 2 mm from contacting the metatarsal head surface (**Fig. 8**). Take care

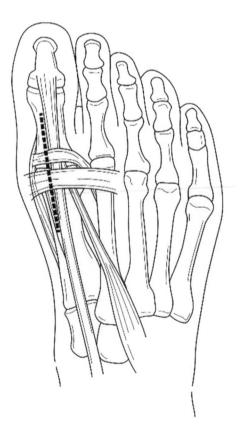

Fig. 3. MTP arthrotomy along the same line of the dorsal incision just medial to the EHL tendon. Dorsal and medial dissection of the joint capsule to allow exposure of the MTP head.

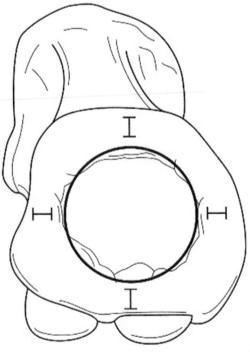

Fig. 4. Minimum of 2 mm of cortical circumferential bone to support radial compression of the synthetic cartilage implant.

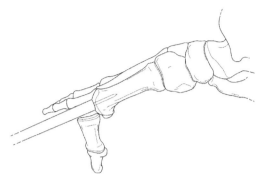

Fig. 5. Concave end of cannulated implant placer on the metatarsal head to allow placement of the guide pin in the central portion of the metatarsal head.

not to compress the reamer step drill bit too firmly against the MT head to avoid making the implantation site too large or deep leading to implant subsidence. Remove the drill bit and guide pin from the implantation site and irrigate to flush out all debris from the reamed hole allowing the implant to seat completely within the bone (Fig. 9).

Step 4

Remove the synthetic cartilage implant from the sterile packaging using smooth forceps and moisten the tapered Introducer Tube with sterile saline. The implant is then inserted into the Introducer Tube with the rounded curved end of the synthetic cartilage implant contacting the plunger and the flat end to the end of the Tube. Firmly grasp the tapered Introducer Tube and put the narrow end firmly against a hard flat sterile operating room surface. Position the small flat end of the Placer against the implant and use your palm to press the wider end of the Placer to advance and compress the implant to the distal end of the Introducer Tube (Fig. 10).

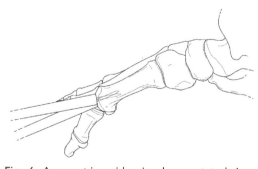

Fig. 6. Asymmetric guide pin placement technique may be used to target synthetic cartilage implantation at the maximum cartilage wear area or the highest point of the MT head.

Step 5

After visualizing that the implant is flush at the end of the Introducer Tube, place the distal end of the Introducer Tube perpendicular to the metatarsal head drill hole, noting that the Introducer Tube will not fit into the metatarsal head cavity. Using your palm and applying careful steady pressure, advance the Placer while maintaining the distal Introducer Tube end precisely at the implant site, to press fit the implant into the metatarsal head. Do not pull back on the Introducer Tube during insertion because this can prevent the base of the implant from being seated flush in the metatarsal head cavity. The implant will be clearly visible following implantation and should be 1.5 to 3 mm proud compared with the adjacent metatarsal head surface to allow for distraction of the joint (Fig. 11).

Step 6

Resect any remaining osteophytes from dorsal, lateral, and medial aspects of metatarsal head again, ensuring there remains a minimum of 2 mm of circumferential cortical rim to support the implant. Confirm range of motion (ROM) of the joint against the implant, checking to make sure there is no restriction or limitation of the joint. Remove all bone debris from the joint and the wound. If there is less dorsiflexion motion than is desired or the proximal phalanx appears in slight plantarflexion that can occur from the chronic contractures of the plantar tissues, a dorsal closing wedge osteotomy of the proximal phalanx can be performed and stabilized with a threaded 0.045 k-wire, staple, or mini-screw if needed. This added phalangeal osteotomy will not alter the postoperative recovery timeline.

Step 7

After irrigation, close the capsule using a 2.0 absorbable suture with standard skin closure and sterile wound dressing. No plaster immobilization is needed. A radiograph of the postoperative implantation is seen in **Figs. 1B and 2B.**

COMPLICATIONS AND MANAGEMENT
Cortical Rim Fracture

If the circumferential cortical rim is fractured, an intraoperative decision is made to determine if the implant remains stable. If implant is not stable, consideration should be given to conversion to a first MTP arthrodesis. This contingency should be discussed with the patient before surgery.

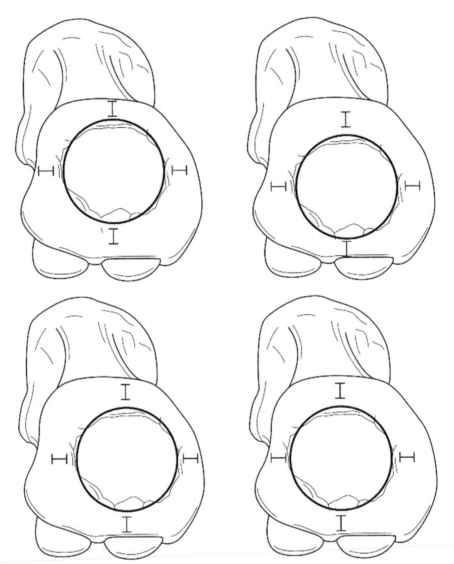

Fig. 7. Irrespective of desired implant position, confirm that a minimum of 2 mm of cortical circumferential bone exists to support the implant.

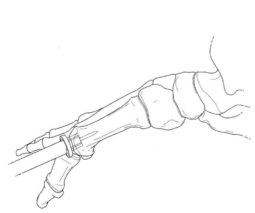

Fig. 8. Ream the MT head until the step drill is 1 to 2 mm from contacting the metatarsal head surface.

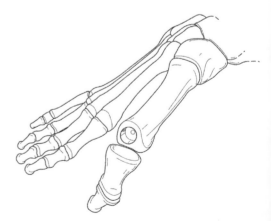

Fig. 9. Guide pin removed and metatarsal cavity cleaned of bone debris to allow proper seating of implant.

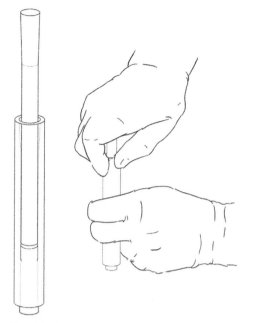

Fig. 10. Compressing implant within the introducer tube, using the placer, on a hard flat sterile, nonshedding surface, in preparation for implantation.

Intraoperative Synthetic Cartilage Implant Recessed Less Than 1.5 mm

If after implantation the implant does not sit 1.5 mm proud, then consideration should be given to removing the implant and adding autologous bone graft potentially from step drill reamings or bone graft substitute to the implantation site base to support the implant. If weak bone at the base of the drill hole is the reason the implant cannot remain proud, packing of additional bone may not provide added support and a first MTP arthrodesis should be considered. If the cause is overreaming of the bone tunnel with the step drill and the base bone of the drill hole is firm, adding bone graft may help. With the addition of this extra bone at the base the implant can be reinserted of synthetic cartilage implant with the goal to have the implant 1.5 to 3 mm proud.

Implant Too Proud

If the implant is more than 3 mm proud after ranging the first MTP joint, the implant can be carefully removed and the guide pin replaced in exactly the same hole to avoid widening the implant tunnel followed by gentle reaming, irrigation, and replacement of the synthetic cartilage implant as outlined above with the goal for implant to be 1.5 to 3 mm proud.

POSTOPERATIVE INSTRUCTIONS

- Compression foot wrap maintaining the first toe in 5° to 10° of dorsiflexion.
- Weight bearing as tolerated (WBAT) in postoperative shoe; no special instructions regarding weight-bearing except to wear protective shoe when ambulating. The patient can sleep without wearing shoe.
- Elevate the foot for the first 5 to 7 days "toes above nose" when sitting.
- Sutures removed at 14 to 21 days postoperatively (Fig. 12).
- The patient is instructed on home ROM exercises (or formal physical therapy if requested) beginning after suture removal and include the following:
  i. Heel rise exercise: Patient instructed to stand and place first toe flat on the floor. Then gently raise their heel off

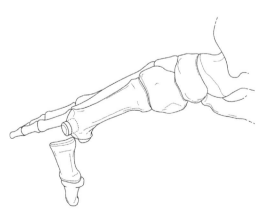

Fig. 11. Implant seated 1.5 to 3 mm proud relative to the surrounding surface following implantation.

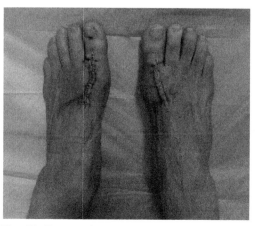

Fig. 12. Two weeks postoperatively, sutures to be removed.

the ground until they feel pressure at the first MTP joint. Continue 10 repetitions with gradual increased dorsiflexion within comfort level. This is performed several times a day if comfortable (Figs. 13 and 14).

   ii. Passive assistive ROM exercise: Patient instructed to gently grasp first toe and passively bring toe upward until they feel stress at the MTP joint. The patient gently grasps the toe plantarly at the proximal phalanx so that they do not stress the interphalangeal (IP) joint. They hold the toe at maximum dorsiflexion for 10 to 20 seconds and then relax. This is repeated 5 times and performed several times a day to comfort (Fig. 15).

- Once sutures are out and patient is working on ROM exercises, they are asked to wean themselves out of the postoperative shoe into sandals or laced shoes accommodating for swelling.
- The patient is advised not to return to fast walking, running, hopping, or toe impact exercises such as soccer for 3 months postoperatively, after which they are recommended to gradually return to these types of activities, but always with a shoe, not a bare foot. A sign of doing "too much" for the patient is if there is pain or swelling with the exercise. If this occurs, the patient needs more recovery time before returning to that higher impact activity.
- Patients are instructed that it could take up to 6 to 12 months for optimal recovery (Table 1).

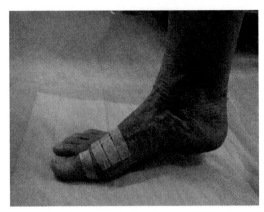

Fig. 14. Heel rise activity loading first MTP joint and keeping proximal phalanx on the floor.

- If additional dorsal closing wedge, phalangeal osteotomy is performed (Moberg osteotomy); the instructions remain the same.

SPECIFIC CLINICAL QUESTIONS

- Do radiographs determine the success or failure of image?
  - Postoperative radiographs do not isolate or detect subsidence due to the spherical nature of the joint. Clinical symptoms of pain over time

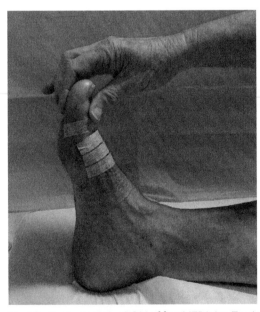

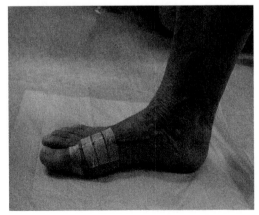

Fig. 13. Lateral clinical photograph of foot after synthetic cartilage implant surgery.

Fig. 15. Passive assistive ROM of first MTP joint. Toe is grasped at the base of proximal phalanx to allow motion to occur through the MTP joint and not the IP joint. The patient holds the dorsiflexion position for 10 to 20 seconds and then relaxes and repeats 5 times.

Table 1
Rehabilitation schedule after synthetic cartilage implant surgery

Weeks 1–2	Elevate foot, walk in compressive dressing and postoperative shoe
Weeks 2+ to 12	Suture removal, home (or formal) physical therapy exercises Wean into sandal or lace-up shoe *Caution: No jumping, running, hopping, or toe impact activities*
12+ wk to 6 mo	Slow progressive return to all activities *Caution: If swelling or pain, allow more time before returning.*
6+ to 12 mo	Continued improvement in pain relief, function and first MTP ROM

(1 year) are an indication for conversion to an arthrodesis.

- Does the patient smoking affect decisions about performing surgery?
  - Like all other orthopedic surgeries, the authors encourage all patients to stop smoking. Current smokers were not excluded from receiving Cartiva implant.
- Is the graft adjusted in patients that choose to wear heels?
  - No, there is no adjustment performed for shoe modification, such as heels.

OUTCOMES

The synthetic cartilage implant has been studied with the only multicentered, prospective randomized study of advanced stage Hallux rigidus with validated outcome measures (pain, function, and motion). In this study, more than 90% of patients with synthetic cartilage implants had significant and clinically meaningful pain relief and improved function while increasing their ROM (average 6°) at 2 years.[9] Approximately 1 in 10 patients had continued pain at 2 years leading to a revision to great toe arthrodesis. After revision to fusion, patients had similar pain relief and functional improvement as if that operation was done primarily, burning no bridges with the implant operation. The 5-year follow-up of the synthetic cartilage implant suggests continued excellent pain relief, function, and maintenance of motion for the 90% of patients who still had the implant in place after 2 years. Recommendations based on this level

1 evidence are that a synthetic cartilage implant is an excellent option for pain and functional improvement in patients with severe hallux rigidus who wish to retain motion. Patients with bunion deformities (hallux valgus >20°) were excluded from this study, and the outcomes cannot be applied to this patient population.

SUMMARY

The synthetic cartilage implant surgery is an excellent option for the patient with great toe arthritis and good alignment of the toe and wishes to retain first MTP motion and obtain significant and clinically meaningful pain relief and improved function, confirmed with rigorous 5-year data. Patients with osteoporosis, osteopenia, or bone defects from surgery or disease may not maintain the implant position because of poor bone quality resulting in less than desired outcomes. Despite this being a straightforward surgery, patients need to be aware that the pain relief may not begin until 3+ months after surgery because this motion-preserving procedure does require bone resection and implant placement. Limitation of functional and sporting activities that load the great toe for 3 months is recommended as well as early motion exercises.

REFERENCES

1. Shereff MJ, Baumhauer JF, et al. Hallux rigidus an osteoarthritis of the first metatarsophalangeal joint. J Bone Joint Surg Am 1998;80(6):898–908.
2. Yee G, Lau J. Current concepts review: hallux rigidus. Foot Ankle Int 2008;29(6):637–46.
3. Gould N, Schneider W, Ashikaga T, et al. Epidemiological survey of foot problems in the continental United States: 1978-1979. Foot Ankle 1980;1(1):8–10.
4. Zammit GV, Menz HB, Munteanu SE, et al. Structural factors associated with hallux limitus/rigidus: a systematic review of case control studies. J Orthop Sports Phys Ther 2009;39(10):733–42.
5. Canseco K, Long J, Marks R, et al. Quantitative characterization of gait kinematics in patients with hallux rigidus using the Milwaukee foot model. J Orthop Res 2008;26(4):419–27.
6. McNeil DS, Baumhauer JF, Glazebrook MA. Evidencebased analysis of the efficacy for operative treatment of hallux rigidus. Foot Ankle Int 2013; 34(1):15–32.
7. Simpson GA, Hembree WC, Miller SD, et al. Surgical strategies: hallux rigidus surgical techniques. Foot Ankle Int 2011;32(12):1175–86.
8. Nollau DFO. SaluCartilage™ Implant—an innovative way for the treatment of osteoarthritis of the

MTP I Joint. Paper presented at American Orthopaedic Foot & Ankle Society (AOFAS) Meeting, La Jolla, California, July 13–16, 2006.

9. Baumhauer JF, Singh D, Glazebrook M, et al. Prospective, randomized, multi-centered clinical trial assessing safety and efficacy of a synthetic cartilage implant versus first metatarsophalangeal

arthrodesis in advanced hallux rigidus. Foot Ankle Int 2016;37(5):457–69.

10. Daniels TR, Younger SE, Penner MJ, et al. Midterm outcomes of polyvinyl alcohol hydrogel hemiarthroplasty of the first metatarsophalangeal joint in advanced hallux rigidus. Foot Ankle Int 2017;38(3): 243–7.

The Use of Tantalum Metal in Foot and Ankle Surgery

Bernard H. Sagherian, MD[a], Richard J. Claridge, MD[b],*

KEYWORDS

- Trabecular metal • Porous tantalum • Structural graft • Bone ingrowth • Foot and ankle
- Arthrodesis • Reconstruction

KEY POINTS

- Several reconstructive procedures in foot and ankle surgery necessitate the use of structural grafts to fill defects, restore height, and maintain correction.
- Autografts are limited in size and volume and can cause substantial donor site morbidity. Allografts, on the other hand, are more readily available; however, they are less osteoinductive and carry the additional risk of disease transmission.
- Tantalum has been used in primary and revision hip and knee replacement surgeries to fill large bony defects and provide support to uncemented components.
- This article is a review of the applications of porous tantalum in foot and ankle surgery.
- Porous tantalum has favorable results in foot and ankle applications and is a viable alternative to the traditional structural grafts without their disadvantages.

BACKGROUND

There are several reconstructive procedures in foot and ankle surgery wherein structural grafts are needed to fill defects, restore height, and maintain correction while providing an osteoconductive environment until fusion occurs.[1–5] These procedures include distraction subtalar arthrodesis, revision of failed subtalar arthrodesis, salvage of failed total ankle arthroplasty, resection for tumor, and various other midfoot fusion procedures.

Traditionally, structural grafts used in foot and ankle arthrodesis procedures have been either autografts or allografts each with its advantages and disadvantages.[1,4–9]

Autografts are limited in their size, and volume can cause substantial donor site morbidity, including numbness, fractures, infection, and pain.[4,10–16] Moreover, harvesting of the autograft might necessitate the use of general anesthesia instead of regional anesthesia alone because of the distance of the donor site from the operative site, as is the case in harvesting tricortical iliac crest graft.

Allografts, on the other hand, do not have associated donor site morbidity. They are readily available and are not significantly limited in size, shape, or volume.[17] However, they are less osteoinductive,[17] with higher rates of nonunion,[18] and carry the additional risk of disease transmission.[19–21] Late collapse with structural failure can be a problem with both autografts and allografts.[22] These limitations can negatively affect the outcome of reconstructive procedures in the foot and ankle. It has been shown that adequately filling the fusion space with graft material is associated with significantly higher fusion rates in

Disclose Statement: B.H. Sagherian has no conflicts of interest. R.J. Claridge is a developer with Zimmer on tantalum spacers since these cases were completed, not at the time these cases were done. He is named on a patent for tantalum spacers.
ᵃ Department of Surgery, Division of Orthopaedic Surgery, American University of Beirut Medical Center, PO Box: 11-0236, Riad El Solh, Beirut 1107 2020, Lebanon; ᵇ Department of Orthopaedic Surgery, Mayo Clinic Arizona, 5777 East Mayo Boulevard, Phoenix, AZ 85054, USA
* Corresponding author.
E-mail address: claridge.richard@mayo.edu

ankle and hindfoot arthrodesis.[23] Another drawback of allografts is the weakening that results from the processing of such grafts. Despite the great advances in fixation techniques to avoid failures and achieve arthrodesis without loss of correction and maintaining structural integrity,[24–28] failures have been reported with both autografts and allografts.

APPLICATION IN ORTHOPEDIC SURGERY

In hip and knee reconstructive surgery, metal augments have replaced the use of large allografts or autografts because of their availability and superior structural integrity. Tantalum has been used in primary and revision hip and knee replacement surgeries to fill large bony defects and provide support to uncemented components.[29–39]

Tantalum has also been used successfully in anterior cervical discectomy and fusion with good radiologic and clinical outcomes. These results have been found to be equivalent to that of autologous grafting and anterior plating, however without the complications of donor site graft harvesting or anterior cervical spine plating.[40,41]

TANTALUM METAL

Tantalum (^{73}Ta) is a dense, hard, highly conductive and chemically stable metal. It has favorable mechanical properties and is a highly corrosion-resistant element. Even highly acidic conditions do not alter its mechanical properties. These characteristics make tantalum a highly inert metal both in vivo and in vitro.[42] Because of its biocompatibility, tantalum has been used safely in several medical fields since the mid-1900s.[42,43] Tantalum-based implants include pacemaker electrodes, foil and mesh for nerve repair, cranioplasty plates, and radiopaque markers.[42,43]

POROUS TANTALUM

Porous tantalum, manufactured for use in orthopedic applications, has a porosity of 80% and pore size ranging from 400 to 600 μm.[44,45] Because of the high volumetric porosity and the nature of interconnecting pores, tantalum is described as a trabecular metal. Trabecular metal is produced through a multistage process that involves the generation of a low-density vitreous carbon skeleton over which pure tantalum is deposited. This vacuum process produces a tantalum coating of 50 μm, which results in a porous tantalum that is 99% tantalum and 1% vitreous carbon in weight.[43,44,46,47] Compared with cobalt chromium and titanium, which are commonly used in orthopedic surgery, porous tantalum has a lower modulus of elasticity, similar to cortical and subchondral bone, and a higher coefficient of friction.[42,44–46] This high coefficient of friction gives porous tantalum substantial initial stability. With stiffness similar to bone, tantalum trabecular metal also prevents stress shielding in the surrounding bone when used in orthopedic applications. The biologic performance of porous tantalum has been well studied. Its biocompatibility and bioactivity with bone ingrowth properties are well established.[46–49] Unlike allograft or autograft bone, which can lose its mechanical properties during or before the bone incorporation process, tantalum trabecular metal retains its mechanical properties because of its fatigue resistance. Because of these properties, porous tantalum has had wide applications in hip and knee reconstructive surgery and more recently in foot and ankle surgery.

Most hip and knee implants are porous coated on the surface. Retrieval studies have shown full-depth penetration of bone into the porous tantalum layer for acetabular shells and femoral stems.[50] Although bone ingrowth at the edges and surfaces should be sufficient for mechanical support, porous tantalum can have the potential of bone incorporation throughout the implant. Bobyn and colleagues[44] have shown in a canine model that by 16 and 52 weeks the average extent of bone ingrowth has ranged from 63% to 80%. Similarly, in a goat model, Sinclair and colleagues[51] have shown bone growth into and around porous tantalum cervical interbody fusion implant margins. They found the open cell porous structure of porous tantalum to facilitate host bone ingrowth and bone bridging through the device, which could be beneficial for long-term mechanical attachment and support in clinical applications.

POROUS TANTALUM IN FOOT AND ANKLE SURGERY

The first report of the use of porous tantalum in foot and ankle was in 2004 by Bouchard and colleagues[52] for tarsometatarsal arthrodesis. The investigators reported sectioning a Trabecular Metal Acetabular Cup (Implex Corporation, Allendale, NJ, USA; Zimmer Inc, Warsaw, IN, USA) and shaping it into 2 wedge-shaped inserts that were used to fill the dorsally based wedge gap. Two separate pieces of tantalum were used to maintain the correction: one on the dorsal aspect of the first tarsometatarsal joint, and the other at the level of the second and the third tarsometatarsal joints. The patient had a solid fusion without any loosening or loss of correction.

Economopoulos and colleagues[53] reported the use of a custom porous tantalum for a distal tibial giant cell tumor in a 43-year-old woman. Computed tomographic (CT) scan was used to determine the dimensions of the porous tantalum. A truncated conical custom porous tantalum spacer measuring 20 mm in length with a centrally open core was fabricated by Zimmer, Inc. Allograft mixed with marrow aspirated from the proximal tibia was packed in the central core. The construct was compressed with screws and a tension band plate. The patient had a solid fusion with painless and unlimited ambulation.

In a pilot study, Frigg and colleagues[54] reported using a tantalum spacer (Zimmer Inc) in 9 patients with complex foot and ankle pathologic conditions. These conditions included a failed revision total ankle replacement, talar osteonecrosis, subtalar nonunion, and severe flatfeet deformities in patients at high risk for failure. The tantalum used was either a spinal fusion device or a cervical fusion device. They reported fusion of all 9 arthrodeses without collapse, loss of correction, or infection and an increase in the American Orthopaedic Foot and Ankle Society (AOFAS) score from a mean of 32 to 74 at the 2-year follow-up. Micro-CT scan was performed on 3 of the 9 patients, which showed condensation of bony trabeculae on the tantalum with bone ingrowth at the bone-implant interface.[54]

Subsequently, Henricson and Rydholm[55] reported on 13 failed total ankle arthroplasties that underwent arthrodesis with the use of a retrograde intramedullary nail through Trabecular Metal Tibial Cones (Zimmer). At a mean of 1.4 years, 7 patients were pain free, 4 had residual pain, however were satisfied with the procedure. None of the patients had radiographic gaps at the bone-implant interface to suggest nonunion.

The largest published series to date is a retrospective review of 27 arthrodesis procedures of the foot and ankle using Trabecular Metal porous tantalum over a period of 5 years.[56] Four patients underwent arthrodesis of the ankle, 17 in the hindfoot, and 6 in the midfoot. The mean age at the time of surgery was 63.1 years and the average follow-up was 27 months. All patients had pathologic conditions that necessitated the use of structural graft. The operative procedures were performed by the senior author (R.J.C.) without modifications from the standard operative techniques except the use Trabecular Metal porous tantalum instead of structural autograft or allograft. The sizes and shapes were custom made for each patient. Pathologic conditions included failed total ankle replacement in 2, posttraumatic ankle arthritis in one, giant cell tumor of the distal tibia in one, posttraumatic hindfoot arthritis in 5, hindfoot arthritis due to tibialis posterior tendon dysfunction in 10, subtalar arthritis due to rheumatoid arthritis in 2, and midfoot arthritis in 6. The porous tantalum was soaked in osteogenic stem cells–rich bone marrow aspirated from the ipsilateral iliac crest. Opteform demineralized bone matrix was used as allograft material to fill any nonstructural defects. The mean AOFAS score improved from 40.6 preoperatively to 86.3 postoperatively. All patients had solid fusion between 4 and 6 months, with absence of lucency at the bone tantalum interface and without loss of correction.[56] Reoperations included removal of painful prominent screws in 3 patients and adjacent joint arthrodesis in one.

Horisberger and colleagues[57] used a Trabecular metal interpositional spacer, specifically designed for tibiotalocalcaneal nailing arthrodesis in 2 patients. The tantalum spacer had a 14-mm hole to allow passage of the retrograde nail. In another report from the same center, Wiewiorski and colleagues[58] used the Trabecular Metal Ankle Fusion Spacer (Zimmer) in conjunction with an anatomic locking compression plate (Synthes, Solothurn, Switzerland).

Sagherian and Claridge[59] have also reported a small series of 3 failed total ankle arthroplasties salvaged by arthrodesis using a tantalum Trabecular Metal (Zimmer) with internal fixation, thus sparing the subtalar joint. Tantalum spacers of the appropriate size were inserted in a press fit manner into and secured with 4.5-mm reconstruction plate in a tension band manner. Small residual defects were packed with Opteform (Exactech, Gainesville, FL, USA) allograft bone mixed with bone marrow aspirated from the ipsilateral iliac crest providing osteogenic elements to enhance healing. The mean age at ankle arthroplasty was 57 years and at ankle arthrodesis was 63 years. Arthrodesis was achieved at a mean of 3 months, and there were no complications.[59]

In a detailed surgical technique for the use of Trabecular metal in tibiocalcaneal arthrodesis, Kreulen and colleagues[60] describe the use of reamer/irrigator/aspirator (RIA) technique (Synthes, West Chester, PA, USA) as an alternative for graft harvesting for use in conjunction with Trabecular Metal spacer in tibiocalcaneal arthrodesis. The RIA is a reaming device with an irrigator and aspirator, which allows harvesting of bone graft from intramedullary canal of long bones, mainly the femur. They accompany this with either Bone Morphogenic Protein-2 or Platelet-Derived Growth Factor. No failures were reported in all 6 patients in their series.

CLINICAL EXAMPLES

Example 1: Distraction Subtalar Arthrodesis

A 67-year-old man, who had sustained a fall from a 6-foot ladder and sustained a left calcaneal fracture, was treated nonoperatively. He had undergone arthrodesis in situ the following year and removal of hardware a year later. The patient was first seen 6 years after the initial injury with lateral hindfoot pain due to fibular impingement (**Fig. 1**). The patient underwent distraction subtalar arthrodesis with a gastrocnemius slide. A tantalum spacer was used measuring 10 mm × 18 mm × 18 mm. At 5-year postoperative follow-up, the patient had a walking tolerance of 2 to 3 miles using regular shoes and with no pain (**Fig. 2**).

Example 2: Salvage of Failed Total Ankle Arthroplasty

A 74-year-old man presented 9 months after a right total ankle arthroplasty with lateral hindfoot pain due to valgus alignment and fibular impingement. Periprosthetic infection was ruled out and a 4-month trial of orthotics with medial wedge improved the symptoms only partially. Surgical treatment included removal of the total ankle arthroplasty and arthrodesis using an off the shelf tantalum augment (**Figs. 3 and 4**). The patient underwent removal of the medial screw 2 years postoperatively due to local pain.

At 8 years postoperatively, the patient had a walking tolerance of 400 yards and was golfing with a cart (**Fig. 5**).

Example 3: Distal Tibial Reconstruction

A 44-year-old woman with giant cell tumor of the right distal tibia presented and had been symptomatic for 1 year before presentation (**Fig. 6**). She underwent excision of the tumor and arthrodesis with a 20-mm conical custom-made tantalum spacer with cancellous autograft (**Fig. 7**). The postoperative course included 6 weeks in a non-weight-bearing cast, another 6 weeks in a weight-bearing removable cast, and 2 years of a custom ankle foot orthosis. At 7 years postoperatively, the patient had a walking tolerance of 1 hour and was using regular shoes (**Figs. 8 and 9**).

Example 4: Calcaneocuboid Distraction Arthrodesis

A 57-year-old woman presented with pain due to equinus deformity and forefoot valgus with collapse of the calcaneocuboid joint of the right foot (**Fig. 10**). The patient underwent distraction calcaneocuboid arthrodesis with 10-mm tantalum spacer, gastrocnemius slide, and first and second tarsometatarsal joint arthrodesis. At 3 years postoperatively, the patient was pain free (**Fig. 11**).

POSTOPERATIVE EVALUATION

Postoperative union was determined based on plain radiographic appearance (absence of lucency at the bone tantalum interface and maintenance of correction) and the clinical absence of pain, tenderness, or swelling.[56] Although CT scan can be a more accurate method for

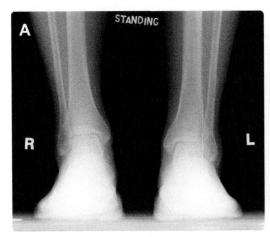
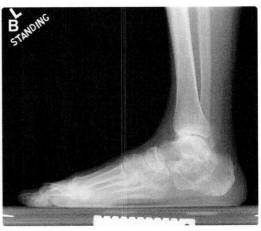

Fig. 1. (*A*, *B*) Radiograph of left ankle status post arthrodesis in situ for a left calcaneal fracture treated nonoperatively initially.

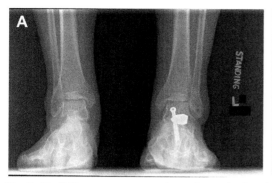
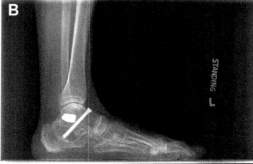

Fig. 2. (A, B) Five-year postoperative radiograph after distraction subtalar arthrodesis using a tantalum spacer.

evaluating subsidence, it does not add much information regarding ingrowth. CT scans have shown intimate contact between the implant and host bone.[53,56]

DISCUSSION

Porous tantalum has emerged as a viable option in reconstructive procedures of the foot and ankle by addressing previous concerns of nonunion and/or loss of correction due to structural graft failure. Most studies using Trabecular Metal for foot and ankle arthrodesis procedures have reported favorable clinical and radiographic outcomes.[52–57,59,60]

Classical structural grafts used include autografts or allografts each with its complications and limitations. Allografts are associated with graft osteolysis and nonunion in up to 50% of cases.[22,61]

Conti and Wong[22] reported 50% failure of calcaneocuboid arthrodesis using an autogenous tricortical iliac crest graft. Reconstructive failure was due to simple nonunion or nonunion with osteolysis and collapse of the graft.

In an attempt to salvage large defects in the ankle, Jeng and colleagues[61] performed tibiocalcaneal arthrodesis using bulk femoral head allografts, either fresh frozen or freeze dried. They reported only 50% fusion rate. Among the fused group, there was a significant 3.6-mm loss of height in the allograft over the 41-month follow-up period. Similar large defects arise after debridement for failed total ankle arthroplasty, which leads to higher rates of complications and nonunions.[5]

Because of the importance of maintaining height during salvage of failed total ankle replacement, Carlsson[62] used a titanium cage filled with autologous bone to fill the defect in 3 patients. None of the ankles healed primarily, and repeat procedures using intramedullary nailing or external fixation was needed. The cages used in this study were meshed titanium alloy cages that were intended to support bone surrounding vertebral defects while harboring cancellous bone grafts; thus the cages did not have a porous surface for potential bone ingrowth. The authors believe that this method works better in spinal surgery due to the

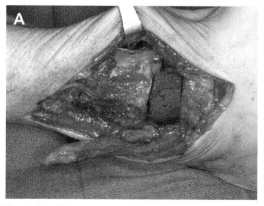
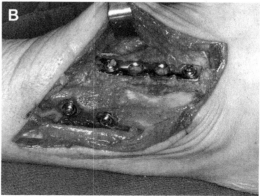

Fig. 3. (A, B) Intraoperative figure demonstrating use of the tantalum spacer to fill the defect after removal of the failed ankle prosthesis.

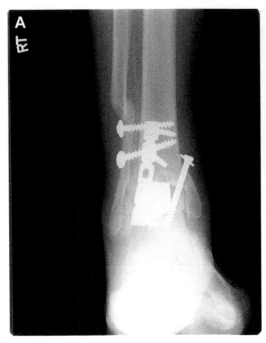
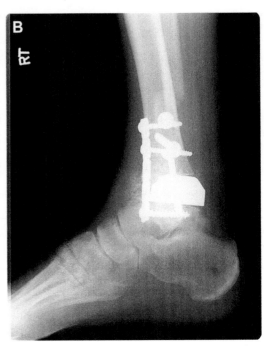

Fig. 4. (*A, B*) Postoperative radiograph of the ankle after arthrodesis using a tantalum spacer for salvage of the failed total ankle arthroplasty.

presence of better cancellous bone and blood flow than in the ankle region, which could be compromised by previous surgery. The authors thus recommended against using this method for ankle arthrodesis.[62] Titanium mesh cages are structurally weaker than block tantalum and therefore not suitable for foot and ankle indications.

An important advantage of porous tantalum is its availability and cost, which is comparable to the cost of allografts. The cost is a compilation of engineering design, manufacturing, and delivery. A detailed cost analysis is beyond

the scope of this article. Suffice to say that the material costs are a small part of the overall cost, so prices are similar for a variety of sizes. Implants are ordered on a custom basis based on the size of the defect and the author's experience. Moreover, its use obviates the operative time needed for autogenous iliac crest graft harvesting, which in turn decreases operative time and operating room fees.

Despite all the reported favorable outcomes, several concerns surround the use of Trabecular Metal. There are no long-term studies regarding

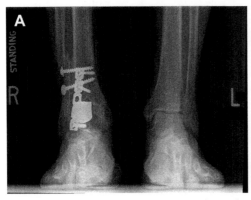
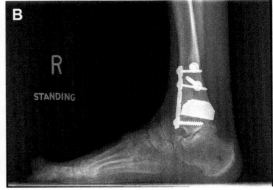

Fig. 5. (*A, B*) Eight-year postoperative radiograph after salvage of the failed total ankle arthroplasty using a tantalum spacer.

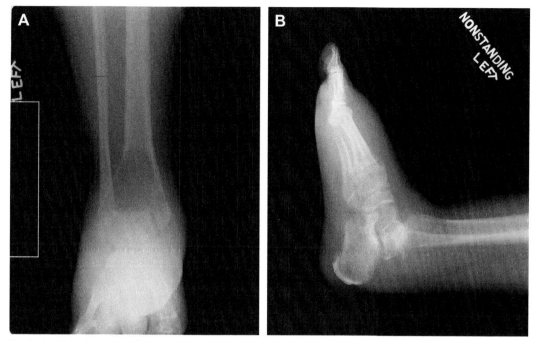

Fig. 6. (*A, B*) Radiograph of the ankle demonstrating changes due to a giant cell tumor.

their application in foot and ankle surgery. Most reports are retrospective reviews, with the largest reported series being 27 patients. A potential disadvantage is the difficulty of removing a well-incorporated tantalum spacer in the case of complications or infections, which might lead to extensive bone loss. Although most Trabecular Metal augments are custom made, modifications in the operating room, if needed, using drills or saws might produce substantial heat that can affect the porosity of the metal and subsequently negatively affect bone ingrowth. To avoid this, tantalum augments and acetabular cups used in hip reconstruction have predrilled holes that can be used for supplementary screw fixation.

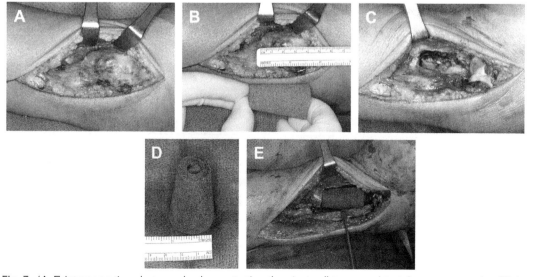

Fig. 7. (*A–E*) Intraoperative photographs demonstrating the giant cell tumor and tantalum spacer used to fill the defect after resection.

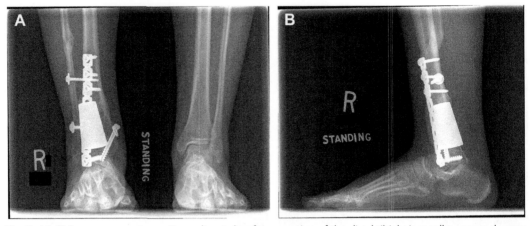

Fig. 8. (A, B) Seven-year postoperative radiographs after resection of the distal tibial giant cell tumor and reconstruction using a tanatalum spacer.

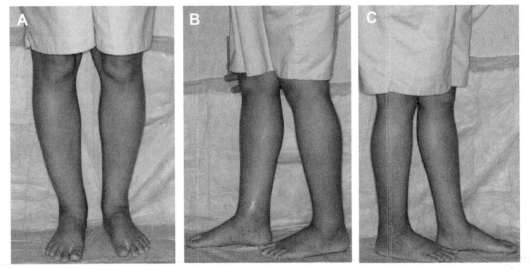

Fig. 9. (A–C) Patient 7 years after the distal tibial giant cell tumor resection and reconstruction using a tantalum spacer.

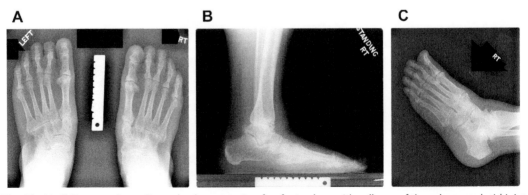

Fig. 10. (A–C) Preoperative radiographs demonstrating forefoot valgus with collapse of the calcaneocuboid joint of the right foot.

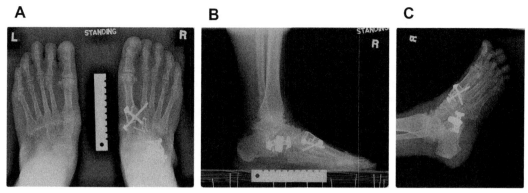

Fig. 11. (A–C) Three-year postoperative radiograph demonstrating distraction calcaneocuboid arthrodesis with tantalum spacer and first and second tarsometatarsal joint arthrodesis.

REFERENCES

1. Chen YJ, Huang TJ, Hsu KY, et al. Subtalar distractional realignment arthrodesis with wedge bone grafting and lateral decompression for calcaneal malunion. J Trauma 1998;45(4):729–37.
2. Horton GA, Olney BW. Triple arthrodesis with lateral column lengthening for treatment of severe planovalgus deformity. Foot Ankle Int 1995;16(7): 395–400.
3. Baumhauer JF, Pinzur MS, Daniels TR, et al. Survey on the need for bone graft in foot and ankle fusion surgery. Foot Ankle Int 2013;34(12):1629–33.
4. Fitzgibbons TC, Hawks MA, McMullen ST, et al. Bone grafting in surgery about the foot and ankle: indications and techniques. J Am Acad Orthop Surg 2011;19(2):112–20.
5. Hopgood P, Kumar R, Wood PL. Ankle arthrodesis for failed total ankle replacement. J Bone Joint Surg Br 2006;88(8):1032–8.
6. Neufeld SK, Uribe J, Myerson MS. Use of structural allograft to compensate for bone loss in arthrodesis of the foot and ankle. Foot Ankle Clin 2002; 7(1):1–17.
7. Amendola A, Lammens P. Subtalar arthrodesis using interposition iliac crest bone graft after calcaneal fracture. Foot Ankle Int 1996;17(10): 608–14.
8. Bednarz PA, Beals TC, Manoli A 2nd. Subtalar distraction bone block fusion: an assessment of outcome. Foot Ankle Int 1997;18(12):785–91.
9. Trnka HJ, Easley ME, Lam PW, et al. Subtalar distraction bone block arthrodesis. J Bone Joint Surg Br 2001;83(6):849–54.
10. Boone DW. Complications of iliac crest graft and bone grafting alternatives in foot and ankle surgery. Foot Ankle Clin 2003;8(1):1–14.
11. Kurz LT, Garfin SR, Booth RE Jr. Harvesting autogenous iliac bone grafts. A review of complications and techniques. Spine 1989;14(12):1324–31.
12. Younger EM, Chapman MW. Morbidity at bone graft donor sites. J Orthop Trauma 1989;3(3):192–5.
13. Heary RF, Schlenk RP, Sacchieri TA, et al. Persistent iliac crest donor site pain: independent outcome assessment. Neurosurgery 2002;50(3):510–6 [discussion: 516–7].
14. Silber JS, Anderson DG, Daffner SD, et al. Donor site morbidity after anterior iliac crest bone harvest for single-level anterior cervical discectomy and fusion. Spine 2003;28(2):134–9.
15. DeOrio JK, Farber DC. Morbidity associated with anterior iliac crest bone grafting in foot and ankle surgery. Foot Ankle Int 2005;26(2):147–51.
16. Arrington ED, Smith WJ, Chambers HG, et al. Complications of iliac crest bone graft harvesting. Clin Orthop Relat Res 1996;(329):300–9.
17. Sammarco VJ, Chang L. Modern issues in bone graft substitutes and advances in bone tissue technology. Foot Ankle Clin 2002;7(1):19–41.
18. Vosseller JT, Ellis SJ, O'Malley MJ, et al. Autograft and allograft unite similarly in lateral column lengthening for adult acquired flatfoot deformity. HSS J 2013;9(1):6–11.
19. Burchardt H. The biology of bone graft repair. Clin Orthop Relat Res 1983;(174):28–42.
20. McGarvey WC, Braly WG. Bone graft in hindfoot arthrodesis: allograft vs autograft. Orthopedics 1996;19(5):389–94.
21. Boyce T, Edwards J, Scarborough N. Allograft bone. The influence of processing on safety and performance. Orthop Clin North Am 1999;30(4): 571–81.
22. Conti SF, Wong YS. Osteolysis of structural autograft after calcaneocuboid distraction arthrodesis for stage II posterior tibial tendon dysfunction. Foot Ankle Int 2002;23(6):521–9.
23. DiGiovanni CW, Lin SS, Daniels TR, et al. The importance of sufficient graft material in achieving foot or ankle fusion. J Bone Joint Surg Am 2016; 98(15):1260–7.

24. Braly WG, Baker JK, Tullos HS. Arthrodesis of the ankle with lateral plating. Foot Ankle Int 1994; 15(12):649–53.

25. Colman AB, Pomeroy GC. Transfibular ankle arthrodesis with rigid internal fixation: an assessment of outcome. Foot Ankle Int 2007;28(3):303–7.

26. Kennedy JG, Hodgkins CW, Brodsky A, et al. Outcomes after standardized screw fixation technique of ankle arthrodesis. Clin Orthop Relat Res 2006; 447:112–8.

27. Maurer RC, Cimino WR, Cox CV, et al. Transarticular cross-screw fixation. A technique of ankle arthrodesis. Clin Orthop Relat Res 1991;(268): 56–64.

28. Tarkin IS, Mormino MA, Clare MP, et al. Anterior plate supplementation increases ankle arthrodesis construct rigidity. Foot Ankle Int 2007;28(2):219–23.

29. Christie MJ. Clinical applications of Trabecular Metal. Am J Orthop (Belle Mead NJ) 2002;31(4): 219–20.

30. Stiehl JB. Trabecular metal in hip reconstructive surgery. Orthopedics 2005;28(7):662–70.

31. Levine B, Della Valle CJ, Jacobs JJ. Applications of porous tantalum in total hip arthroplasty. J Am Acad Orthop Surg 2006;14(12):646–55.

32. Levine B, Sporer S, Della Valle CJ, et al. Porous tantalum in reconstructive surgery of the knee: a review. J Knee Surg 2007;20(3):185–94.

33. Unger AS, Lewis RJ, Gruen T. Evaluation of a porous tantalum uncemented acetabular cup in revision total hip arthroplasty: clinical and radiological results of 60 hips. J Arthroplasty 2005;20(8): 1002–9.

34. Meneghini RM, Lewallen DG, Hanssen AD. Use of porous tantalum metaphyseal cones for severe tibial bone loss during revision total knee replacement. J Bone Joint Surg Am 2008;90(1):78–84.

35. Sporer SM, Paprosky WG. The use of a trabecular metal acetabular component and trabecular metal augment for severe acetabular defects. J Arthroplasty 2006;21(6 Suppl 2):83–6.

36. Long WJ, Scuderi GR. Porous tantalum cones for large metaphyseal tibial defects in revision total knee arthroplasty: a minimum 2-year follow-up. J Arthroplasty 2009;24(7):1086–92.

37. Kamath AF, Lewallen DG, Hanssen AD. Porous tantalum metaphyseal cones for severe tibial bone loss in revision knee arthroplasty: a five to nine-year follow-up. J Bone Joint Surg Am 2015; 97(3):216–23.

38. Brown NM, Bell JA, Jung EK, et al. The use of trabecular metal cones in complex primary and revision total knee arthroplasty. J Arthroplasty 2015;30(9 Suppl):90–3.

39. Sheth NP, Lonner JH. Clinical use of porous tantalum in complex primary total knee arthroplasty. Am J Orthop (Belle Mead NJ) 2009;38(10):526–30.

40. Fernandez-Fairen M, Sala P, Dufoo M Jr, et al. Anterior cervical fusion with tantalum implant: a prospective randomized controlled study. Spine 2008;33(5):465–72.

41. Fernandez-Fairen M, Murcia A, Torres A, et al. Is anterior cervical fusion with a porous tantalum implant a cost-effective method to treat cervical disc disease with radiculopathy? Spine 2012; 37(20):1734–41.

42. Black J. Biological performance of tantalum. Clin Mater 1994;16(3):167–73.

43. Cohen R. A porous tantalum trabecular metal: basic science. Am J Orthop (Belle Mead NJ) 2002;31(4):216–7.

44. Bobyn JD, Stackpool GJ, Hacking SA, et al. Characteristics of bone ingrowth and interface mechanics of a new porous tantalum biomaterial. J Bone Joint Surg Br 1999;81(5):907–14.

45. Levine BR, Sporer S, Poggie RA, et al. Experimental and clinical performance of porous tantalum in orthopedic surgery. Biomaterials 2006;27(27):4671–81.

46. Shimko DA, Shimko VF, Sander EA, et al. Effect of porosity on the fluid flow characteristics and mechanical properties of tantalum scaffolds. J Biomed Mater Res B Appl Biomater 2005;73(2): 315–24.

47. Zardiackas LD, Parsell DE, Dillon LD, et al. Structure, metallurgy, and mechanical properties of a porous tantalum foam. J Biomed Mater Res 2001; 58(2):180–7.

48. Kokubo T, Kim HM, Kawashita M. Novel bioactive materials with different mechanical properties. Biomaterials 2003;24(13):2161–75.

49. Welldon KJ, Atkins GJ, Howie DW, et al. Primary human osteoblasts grow into porous tantalum and maintain an osteoblastic phenotype. J Biomed Mater Res A 2008;84(3):691–701.

50. Hanzlik JA, Day JS. Bone ingrowth in well-fixed retrieved porous tantalum implants. J Arthroplasty 2013;28(6):922–7.

51. Sinclair SK, Konz GJ, Dawson JM, et al. Host bone response to polyetheretherketone versus porous tantalum implants for cervical spinal fusion in a goat model. Spine 2012;37(10):E571–80.

52. Bouchard M, Barker LG, Claridge RJ. Technique tip: tantalum: a structural bone graft option for foot and ankle surgery. Foot Ankle Int 2004;25(1): 39–42.

53. Economopoulos K, Barker L, Beauchamp C, et al. Case report: reconstruction of the distal tibia with porous tantalum spacer after resection for giant cell tumor. Clin Orthop Relat Res 2010;468(6): 1697–701.

54. Frigg A, Dougall H, Boyd S, et al. Can porous tantalum be used to achieve ankle and subtalar arthrodesis?: a pilot study. Clin Orthop Relat Res 2010;468(1):209–16.

55. Henricson A, Rydholm U. Use of a trabecular metal implant in ankle arthrodesis after failed total ankle replacement. Not Found In Database 2010;81(6): 745–7.

56. Sagherian BH, Claridge RJ. Porous tantalum as a structural graft in foot and ankle surgery. Foot Ankle Int 2012;33(3):179–89.

57. Horisberger M, Paul J, Wiewiorski M, et al. Commercially available trabecular metal ankle interpositional spacer for tibiotalocalcaneal arthrodesis secondary to severe bone loss of the ankle. J Foot Ankle Surg 2014;53(3):383–7.

58. Wiewiorski M, Schlemmer T, Horisberger M, et al. Ankle fusion with a trabecular metal spacer and an anterior fusion plate. J Foot Ankle Surg 2015; 54(3):490–3.

59. Sagherian BH, Claridge RJ. Salvage of failed total ankle replacement using tantalum trabecular metal: case series. Foot Ankle Int 2015;36(3): 318–24.

60. Kreulen C, Lian E, Giza E. Technique for use of trabecular metal spacers in tibiotalocalcaneal arthrodesis with large bony defects. Foot Ankle Int 2017;38(1):96–106.

61. Jeng CL, Campbell JT, Tang EY, et al. Tibiotalocalcaneal arthrodesis with bulk femoral head allograft for salvage of large defects in the ankle. Foot Ankle Int 2013;34(9):1256–66.

62. Carlsson A. Unsuccessful use of a titanium mesh cage in ankle arthrodesis: a report on three cases operated on due to a failed ankle replacement. J Foot Ankle Surg 2008;47(4):337–42.

Technologies in the Treatment of Bone Marrow Edema Syndrome

Reza A. Ghasemi, MD*, Saleh Sadeghi, MD,
Narges Rahimee, MD, Mohamadnaghi Tahmasebi, MD

KEYWORDS

• BMES • Transient osteoporosis • Iloprost • Bisphosphonate • Core decompression

KEY POINTS

- Bone marrow edema syndrome (BMES) is a rare and self-limited syndrome with an unknown cause.
- The natural time course for improvement of clinical symptoms and normalization in MRI lasts from 3 to 18 months.
- This entity must be distinguished from other causes of marrow abnormality, such as stress fractures and osteonecrosis, for the best treatment options.
- Various treatments from conservative to surgical have been made to provide pain relief and to accelerate the natural course of the disease.
- The purpose of this article is to review BMES with a focus on treatment in the foot and ankle.

INTRODUCTION

Bone marrow edema syndrome (BMES) is a rare and self-limited syndrome characterized by disabling bone pain and increased interstitial fluid within the bone marrow without a definable cause.[1–3] BMES initially was defined in 1959 as a clinical syndrome characterized by hip pain and decreased bone density on radiographs during the last trimester of pregnancy.[4] The most common sites involved in BMES are the hip, knee, ankle, and foot bones.[5,6] Because of the low prevalence and unspecific symptoms, the correct diagnosis often is delayed. This delay may aggravate bone pain and impairs function and quality of life.[7] Hence, the syndrome may be misdiagnosed and treated incorrectly for other conditions, such as osteonecrosis.[1,8] The aim of this article is to increase awareness among orthopedic surgeons about the current treatment options for BMES with a focus on treatment in the foot and ankle.

ETIOLOGY

The cause of BMES of the foot and ankle is still unclear. However, it has been suggested low systemic bone mineral density caused by vitamin D deficiency may be associated with BMES.[6] Furthermore, some investigations reported an association between BMES and pregnancy (especially the last trimester), microtrauma (overuse injuries), type IV hyperlipoproteinemia, cirrhosis, and electromyographic abnormalities.[2,9–12] Bone marrow edema risk factors include corticosteroid therapy, sickle cell anemia, alcohol and nicotine abuse, trauma, rheumatic diseases, fat metabolism disorders, radiotherapy, and chemotherapy. The major risk factor for bone marrow edema in the foot and ankle is microtrauma.[5,9]

DIAGNOSIS

Most patients who have BMES report severe and disabling pain that severely limits activities of

Tehran University of Medical Science, Number 21, Dameshgh Street, Vali-e Asr Avenue, Tehran 1416753955, Iran
* Corresponding author. 1300 Fayette Street, Apartment 2, Conshohocken, PA 19428.
E-mail address: ghasemiar2@gmail.com

Orthop Clin N Am 50 (2019) 131–138
https://doi.org/10.1016/j.ocl.2018.08.008

daily living.[1,6] The definitive diagnosis of BMES is made with the clinical examination and MRI scan; changes on MRI scan (decreased signal intensity on T1-weighted images and increased signal intensity on T2-weighted images) may be observed within 48 hours after onset of symptoms.[13,14] Laboratory results usually are normal in patients with BMES including complete blood counts, electrolytes, alkaline phosphatase, antinuclear antibody, erythrocyte sedimentation rate, C-reactive protein, and rheumatoid factor. In some cases, a mild elevated erythrocyte sedimentation rate has been noted.[2,7,13] In addition, hypovitaminosis D may be associated with BMES of the foot and ankle, and assessment of vitamin D levels and treatment of bone mineral density is suggested.[6]

PATHOPHYSIOLOGY AND HISTOLOGY

The pathogenesis of BMES is poorly understood. Possible theories suggested include changes in lipid metabolism, abnormalities of vascular factors, such as thrombocyte aggregation; thromboembolism; decreased antithrombin III level; decreased fibrinolysis in pregnant women with increase in plasminogen activator inhibitor 1 or lipoprotein levels; occlusion of arteriolar or venous flow; or damaged blood vessel walls caused by vasculitis.[15–18] The pain in BMES could be caused by irritation or disruption of sensory nerves within the bone marrow. Sensory nerve irritation is caused by an increase intraosseous pressure from 20 to 30 mm Hg to 50 to 90 mm Hg, and sensory nerve disruption is caused by tumors or trauma that may cause disruption of capillary leakage.[14,19] Another possible mechanism suggested for the pathogenesis of BMES includes proximal nerve root ischemia caused BMES pain from denervation.[20]

TREATMENT
Symptomatic Treatment
The aims of BMES treatment are to decrease the clinical course and relieve pain (Table 1). Generally, BMES improves within 3 to 9 months without treatment. Symptomatic treatment usually includes off-loading or pharmacologic treatment.[6,7,13,21,22] Preliminary studies of BMES represented no beneficial effects of treatment with antituberculosis drugs, prednisone, calcitonin, or lumbar sympathectomy.[23] Further treatments that have been related to pain reduction in limited patients who have BMES include sympathetic nerve blockade with bupivacaine (in three patients, in whom pathologic recovery was not observed on MRI scans) and nifedipine (in a short review).[24,25]

Symptomatic nonoperative treatment involves nonsteroidal anti-inflammatory drugs (NSAIDs), partial weightbearing or nonweightbearing, removable walker boot, calcium, physiotherapy, and massage therapy, and may need 6 to 12 months for complete recovery.[3,6,8,23,26] However, this regimen may not be accepted by professional athletes who need rapid return to competition and daily activities.[27]

Iloprost
Since 1998 the drug iloprost, a synthetic analogue of prostacyclin, has been registered for the treatment of early stages of osteonecrosis and BMES.[28] In addition, iloprost has been applied for the treatment of critical ischemia secondary to peripheral atherosclerotic diseases or diabetic angiopathy. It causes arterial and venous dilation and improves microcirculation by acting on rheologic properties of the terminal vascular bed, reduction in capillary permeability, inhibition of platelet aggregation, improving the viscosity of distal vessels, and decreasing oxygen free radicals and leukotrienes concentration.[15,29]

G-protein coupling with the prostanoid receptor represents an important role in mediating the effects of prostacyclin. Activation of prostacyclin receptors may result in inflammatory responses, pain sensation, inhibition of thrombocyte aggregation, and vasodilation. In addition, prostacyclin (PGI_2) is a main mediator in bone metabolism and remodeling, which acts via the kinase A-pathway as a potent inhibitor of bone resorption.[30] Iloprost primarily is administered in the treatment of pulmonary hypertension, ischemia, scleroderma, and Buerger disease.[5] Other rare indications for iloprost include severe bone pain caused by sickle cell crisis, systemic lupus erythematosus, and Raynaud phenomenon. Furthermore, iloprost improves organ storage and preservation of liver, lung, heart, and kidney transplant.[30] Iloprost is contraindicated in patients with heart failure; gastrointestinal ulcers; myocardial infarction or recent unstable angina; pregnancy and breastfeeding period; and treatment with anticoagulant drugs, such as warfarin or heparin.[16] Iloprost therapy has been assessed in patients with BMES in the foot and ankle. In a study of 10 patients with BMES of the foot and ankle who were treated with iloprost (intravenous administration for 5–6 hours on 5 consecutive days; iloprost dose: first day, 20 μg; second day, 30 μg; third to fifth day, 40 μg; drug dose decreased by 20 μg for adverse effects), pain was immediately decreased after the first few days of treatment. The MRI scan at 1-year follow-up after therapy

Table 1
Treatment options in studies of bone marrow edema syndrome

Treatment Options		Mean Treatment Duration	Mean Improvement Duration
Symptomatic treatment	Off-loading (non/partial weightbearing) Nonsteroidal anti-inflammatory drugs Physiotherapy	Undefinable duration	6–12 mo
Prostacyclins	Iloprost	5 consecutive days	After treatment (d/wk)
Bisphosphonates	Alendronate	Several weeks	After months
	Ibandronate	1–3 doses at monthly intervals	Rapid pain free
	Denosumab	Single dose	After treatment (days)
	Zolendronic acid	Undefinable duration	After months
Pulsed electromagnetic fields	Pulsed electromagnetic field stimulation	1 mo (daily)	After treatment (1 mo)
Vitamin D	Correcting serum vitamin D levels by using vitamin D supplements should be assessed		
Polysulfated polysaccharides	Pentosan polysulfate	It can resolve the clinical symptoms and diminish the size of the bone marrow edema, when such a treatment is required	
Surgical treatments	Subchondroplasty Core decompression	It may be considered after conservative treatment of rapid and complete reduction of symptoms	

in seven patients showed reduction of bone marrow edema in six patients.[29] In another study of 23 patients with BMES of the foot and ankle, iloprost treatment was given for 5 days (0.5 ng/kg/min >6 h/d intravenous administration). After treatment, the patients were partial weightbearing (≤15 kg) for 6 weeks. Current study represents improvement in functional outcomes in addition to complete regression of edema, which is deduced from MRI at third month following treatment in 22 out of 23 patients.[5] Another study evaluated 19 patients with iloprost administrations (50 µg; in some patients, 20 µg to minimize adverse events). Most patients who suffered side effects had been treated with 50-µg infusion. Pain at rest was relieved after 5 days, and pain during activity was relieved after 3 weeks. Follow-up MRI scan at 3 months after therapy showed complete remission of edema in most patients.[27] In other studies, infusion of iloprost (40 or 50 µg) in 500 mL sodium chloride solution for more than 6 h/d and 5 days showed similar results.[1,15,31] Adverse effects with iloprost may be minor or severe. Severe side effects may include arrhythmia, bleeding, hypotension, thromboembolism, acute respiratory distress

syndrome, pulmonary edema, and allergic reactions resulting in clinical signs of systemic shock. Minor side effects include headache, nausea, flushing, erythema, and phlebitis.[30,32] Treatment of common side effects, such as nausea, headache, flulike syndrome, cough, flushing, or insomnia, may include brief interruption of treatment, dose reduction, analgesic drugs, and antiemetic drugs.[5,15]

Bisphosphonates

Increased bone turnover in BMES proposes that bisphosphonates may be beneficial in the treatment.[7] These class of drugs are strong antiresorptive (anticatabolic) agents that act on intracellular components of the mevalonate pathway and inhibit the prenylation of intracellular proteins in osteoclasts. Bisphosphonate therapy may cause revascularization and bone formation.[29] Pamidronate (intravenous), clodronate (intravenous), and alendronate (oral) have been applied successfully in patients with bone marrow edema. Pamidronate and clodronate need prolonged slow intravenous administration to prevent renal toxicity and must be applied in a hospital, which may be difficult, expensive, unpleasant, and associated with complications.[33]

Alendronate

Alendronate is approved and commonly used to treat bone loss in adults. Oral alendronate provides some clinical advantages to administration by intravenous infusion, but it must be given frequently with strict dosing. Having to follow-up daily or weekly dosing guidelines is inconvenient and may delay therapy compliance. In addition, poor enteral absorption may be delayed with oral dosing in achieving a clinical response.[33] In a study that included 18 patients with BMES of the foot and ankle, symptomatic treatment included pneumatic walker boot for 8 weeks in all patients. Pain improved in seven patients within 26 weeks. The other 11 patients who did not have improvement during follow-up for 8 weeks were treated with one infusion of zolendronic acid (5 mg; nine patients) or weekly oral alendronate (two patients, because of complications with intravenous bisphosphonates). The patients had relief of symptoms within mean 16 weeks after oral and 5.8 weeks after intravenous treatment.[3]

Ibandronate

Ibandronate, a nitrogen-containing bisphosphonate, has been proven in relieving pain in malignant disorders. Unlike current intravenous bisphosphonates, ibandronate may be administered by rapid intravenous injection rather than prolonged infusion and this may be performed with high-dose intervals (once every 2–3 months).[33] Therefore, intravenous ibandronate for outpatient treatment of BMES may be a safe, effective, and economical option.[7] Therapy with ibandronate for BMES of the foot and ankle has been assessed in several studies. In a study of two patients with foot and ankle BMES, treatment included one dose of ibandronate (4 mg intravenous), an optional second dose (2 mg) after 3 months, calcium (1 g daily), and vitamin D (800 IU daily); the patients had rapid pain free and returned to work at 4 weeks after start of treatment.[33] In another study seven high-performance athletes with BMES of the foot and ankle were treated with ibandronate (3 mg intravenous), calcium (600 mg daily), and vitamin D (400 IU daily). Earlier diagnosis and onset of treatment resulted in earlier return to competition (diagnosis within 40 days: return to competition, 64 ± 48 d; later diagnosis: return to competition, 124 ± 63 d; $P \leq .05$). Vitamin D and calcium supplements were considered important to reduce the risk of hypocalcemia. In patients who had no clinical improvement after the first dose of ibandronate and no reduction in bone marrow edema on MRI scan,

additional ibandronate (1 or 2 doses) was taken.[28] In a previous study, 15 patients with ankle BMES were assessed in two groups and treated with or without off-loading (nonweight-bearing for 3 weeks, then partial weightbearing for 3 weeks), analgesics (diclofenac sodium, 150 mg/d for 3 weeks), and ibandronate infusions (each infusion, 6 mg in 100 mL sodium chloride over 30 minutes; three ambulatory infusions at monthly intervals). Patients who received ibandronate had considerably better outcomes including improved functional scores, performance of daily activities, working ability, and reduced amount of bone marrow edema on MRI scans.[7] Adverse events of ibandronate include flulike symptoms, osteonecrosis of the jaw, acute phase reaction, muscle pain, uveitis, nephrocalcinosis, and renal failure.[7,29] Contraindications to ibandronate include pregnancy, hypocalcemia, severe chronic kidney disease, or history of jaw osteonecrosis.[28] In a recent study, patients had renal function blood tests and ultrasonography before treatment because of concerns about possible renal complications. In addition, total serum calcium level was measured on the first and third days after starting bisphosphonate infusion because of the risk of hypocalcemia, and patients were followed every 3 months to monitor for rare complications of bisphosphonates, such as uveitis and osteonecrosis of the jaw.[29]

Denosumab

Denosumab is a human monoclonal antibody for the treatment of osteoporosis. It acts by binding to RANKL to inhibit its interaction with RANK receptors on osteoclasts and decreases bone resorption. Denosumab has been revealed to decrease remodeling more effectively and more quickly than bisphosphonates. Because bone marrow edema may develop rapidly, denosumab might be a better and more potent agent because of its superior skeletal distribution and more rapid inhibition of osteoclasts. Bone resorption reduced considerably after denosumab administration, whereas bone formation was decreased concordantly indicating a decrease in bone turnover. This effect illustrates the mechanism of drug action. Furthermore, a balanced calcium and vitamin D homeostasis has been found to be necessary before the administration of an antiresorptive treatment. Therefore, patients suffering from BMES should be treated with adequate dose vitamin D before and after denosumab administration. Overall, denosumab injection seems to be safe, although calcium serum levels have to be checked for hypocalcemia before treatment in all patients and after treatment in patients with compromised renal function.[34,35] In a retrospective study (level of evidence 3) including 14 symptomatic patients with BMES, the affected skeletal sites were femoral head (n = 8), distal femur (n = 5), and metatarsals (n = 1). The patients were treated with 200,000 IE vitamin D weekly before the denosumab application. The injection included a single dose of subcutaneous denosumab, 60 mg. MRI scans were done before and 6 to 12 weeks after the denosumab treatment. The bone marrow edema ameliorated completely in 50% of patients 6 to 12 weeks after denosumab therapy and was reduced in an additional six patients, although it remained constant in only one patient and worsened in no cases. This study indicates an overall treatment success of 93% and a treatment success of 78.5% not including the patients with additional core decompression. VAS score (Visual Analog Score) decreased significantly between initial presentation and postintervention. The treatment was well tolerated in all 14 patients with no side effects.[35]

Zoledronic Acid

Zolendronic acid is a highly potent bisphosphonate that inhibits bone resorption and osteoclastic activity. It can also block the osteoclastic resorption of mineralized bone and skeletal calcium release through its binding to bone. In a study that included 17 patients diagnosed with BMES who had been refractory to standard treatments (reduced weight-bearing and NSAIDs) in the previous 2 to 3 months, patients were treated with zoledronic acid. The most frequently affected joint was the foot and ankle (nine patients), followed by the hip. Of those patients, 13 had no pain after 12 months. Follow-up MRIs were available in 8 out of 17 patients; five represented edema disappearance in the MRI. As for the three remaining patients, a reduction of the initial edema by more than 50% could be observed in the images. No severe adverse effects attributed to zoledronic acid administration were reported during follow-up.[36]

Vitamin D

Vitamin D deficiency is a worldwide health concern, and recently it is estimated that this vitamin affects more than 1 billion people in the world. Hence, it is not unexpected that vitamin D is also frequently insufficient in orthopedic patients. Because the reason of BMES is still unidentified, presently no generally accepted guideline exists for the treatment of BMES of the foot and ankle. Lately, it has become obvious that BMES occurs along with an increment in bone turnover. It is well identified that vitamin D is a key element to maintain balanced bone turnover and a healthy bone microenvironment. More recently, numerous studies showed that untreated hypovitaminosis D not only causes well-known diseases, such as osteoporosis, rickets, and osteomalacia, but also shows several other osseous impacts. Singularly, low vitamin D levels are related to an increment in numerous chronic and infectious diseases and aggravation of many orthopedic disease arrangements.[34,37] In a study, 31 patients were identified with BMES of the foot and ankle. The diagnosis was based on the clinical check, the presence of abnormal bone marrow signal intensity in T1- and T2-weighted MRI, the existence of prolonged foot pain, and the patient's medical history. Remarkably, 84% of patients (26/31) were with low vitamin D levels and a mean 25(OH)D level of 19.03 ng/mL. Specifically, 61% of patients (19/31) had vitamin D–deficient levels, 23% (7/31) vitamin D–insufficient levels, and only 16% of patients (5/31) had sufficient vitamin D levels. In this study, a high rate of hypovitaminosis D was found and vitamin D deficiency among patients was diagnosed with BMES of the foot and ankle. Therefore, they consider that inadequate vitamin D levels might be a key cofactor in the development and course of the disease. Vitamin D supplementation is simple and safe; therefore, correcting serum vitamin D levels through use of vitamin D supplements might impact on the development and course of BMES of the foot.[37]

Pulsed Electromagnetic Fields

It was reported that treatment with pulsed electromagnetic fields (PEFs) produces anti-inflammatory and bone-healing effects, hence reducing the production of free radicals and stimulating the osteogenic activity of osteoblasts. It seems that PEF treatment of bone marrow edema with increased bone turnover decreases the pain by removing the bone marrow edema and shortening the natural course of the disease. Previous studies indicated that PEF stimulation may have a role in the further treatment of cartilaginous pathologic abnormalities. An anti-inflammatory effect accompanied by decreased production of free radicals is induced, increasing the availability of the A2A adenosine receptors placed on the membrane of neutrophils. It prevents catabolic impacts of inflammatory cytokines (ie, interleukin-1) on the joint cartilage and motivates the synthesis of proteo-glycans; in addition, it bounds the progression of osteoarthritis in vivo, inducing cytokine expression with anabolic effects on cartilage and preventing the expression of cytokines with catabolic impacts. Moreover, treatment with PEF reduced the use of NSAIDs and improved functional recovery. Treatment with PEFs indicated obvious advantages concerning costs, risks, and potential adverse effects in comparison with the intravenous administration of iloprost or ibandronate.[38,39] In a study, this novel conservative approach was evaluated to treat bone marrow edema of the talus using PEFs to investigate safety and potential effect measures. In the study, six patients with bone marrow edema of the talus diagnosed by MRI were involved. In all of the patients, previous treatment included NSAIDs, physical therapy in four of the six patients, and weight-bearing reduction in the other two, with no substantial impact on their symptoms. Treatment involved PEF stimulation 8 h/d, continuous for 30 days. An MRI test was conducted to investigate treatment efficiency at follow-up visits (ie, every month) until edema resolution. Five patients reported significant improvement following 1 month of treatment, and one patient with residual pain followed PEF therapy for 30 days, with whole pain relief at the second follow-up visit. At the last follow-up (mean, 10.8 months; range, 7–14 months), the mean American Orthopedic Foot and Ankle Society score enhanced from 59.4 (range, 40–66) before treatment to 94 (range, 80–100). There was a significant reduction in visual analog scale score from 5.6 (range, 4–7) before treatment to 1 (range, 0–2) at the last follow-up.[39]

Polysulfated Polysaccharides

Polysulfated polysaccharide was recently described as an effective treatment of bone marrow edema. Heparin and structurally related polysulfated polysaccharides, such as chitosan polysulfate and pentosan polysulfate (PPS), were used as anticoagulants for some years. PPS is a weaker anticoagulant compared with heparin; however, it has been used as a thrombolytic agent prophylactically and postsurgically. PPS has also been recommended as a disease-modifying drug for osteoarthritis. Moreover, using it, symptomatic relief was demonstrated in patients with osteoarthritis. It has been revealed that polysulfated polysaccharides or PPS distributed systemically or orally to a patient with bone marrow edema can improve clinical symptoms and decrease the size of bone marrow edema. It has also been demonstrated that polysulfated

polysaccharides can diminish local tumor necrosis factor-α produced by bone marrow edema cells, which are assumed to be the initial mediator of cellular and vascular changes promoting the pain. Consequently, this patent involves a method for the treatment of bone marrow edema by administering an effective amount of a polysulfated polysaccharide when such a treatment is required.[40] However, data about this method in patients who have BMES have not been reported and further clinical studies are needed to elucidate the uncertainties concerning the relative effectiveness of polysulfated polysaccharides in BMES.

SURGICAL TREATMENT

There are few literature-recommend surgical treatments of BMES, possibly because BMES is self-limited and conservative treatments usually have satisfactory results. Surgical treatment that has been proposed includes core decompression and subchondroplasty.

Core Decompression

Although few cases are treated with core decompression, it may be considered for rapid and complete reduction of symptoms and improvement of MRI changes. In addition, core decompression has low morbidity and is an outpatient procedure, but the procedure requires partial weightbearing and physiotherapy. The reported pain relief after core decompression method (drilling a hole in the involved area leads to reduce pressure and allows for increasing blood supply) supports the theory that BMES pain may be caused by increased intramedullary pressure.[13,15,41] In a study of 10 patients with BMES of the foot, core decompression was performed in four patients after conservative treatment and provided rapid relief of symptoms; the other six patients who were treated with limited weightbearing and analgesics had considerable delay in pain reduction.[13] In another report of a 45-year-old woman with BMES of the foot, core decompression of the navicular bone was performed. One week after operative treatment, the patient had no pain and MRI scan at 3 months after surgery revealed complete recovery of abnormal signal intensity.[42]

Subchondroplasty

Injection of calcium phosphate was observed as a potentially viable treatment option. To describe the technique of injecting a flowable calcium phosphate synthetic bone-void filler into the space between the trabeculae of cancellous bone in the subchondral region the term subchondroplasty is used. The calcium phosphate experiences an endothermic reaction while imitating the strength and porosity of normal cancellous bone. Over the next several months, osteoclasts or osteoblasts can use this scaffold-like implant to remodel local bone.[43–45] In a case study, the patient was treated conservatively for plantar fasciitis involving steroid injections, night splints, physical therapy, and orthotics. However, conservative treatments failed to provide her constant pain relief for her daily activities and an MRI was acquired. The results of the MRI indicated plantar fasciitis with faint primary bone marrow edema. When conservative care is not effective, surgical intervention is warranted. Open and endoscopic plantar fasciotomies have documented achievement rates of 76% in these recalcitrant patients. However, this case with continued pain and disability failed conservative and initial surgical intervention. The enlarged presence of calcaneal bone marrow edema on her follow-up MRI forced them to try an innovative method for using subchondroplasty along with revision fasciotomy. Nine months following the calcaneal subchondroplasty, the patient felt no pain and could run. In those patients with identifiable bone marrow lesions on MRI with continued pain, this surgical treatment should be assessed as an adjunctive procedure.[15]

SUMMARY

BMES is a rare entity that should be distinguished from other causes of marrow abnormality for appropriate patient management. MRI scan is the most valuable tool for definitive diagnosis of BMES. Conservative to surgical approaches have been assessed so far for BMES. Notwithstanding, it is difficult to identify the best strategy. Conservative treatments including symptomatic and pharmacologic treatments are typically the preferable alternatives because of satisfactory therapeutic response. Surgical treatment may be considered in patients with refractory pain and rapid reduction of symptoms. Complementary measures, such as assessment and repletion of serum vitamin D and calcium, should be recommended.

REFERENCES

1. Arazi M, Yel M, Uguz B, et al. Be aware of bone marrow edema syndrome in ankle arthroscopy: a case successfully treated with iloprost. Arthroscopy 2006;22(8):909.e1-3.

2. Gigena LM, Chung CB, Lektrakul N, et al. Transient bone marrow edema of the talus: MR imaging findings in five patients. Skeletal Radiol 2002;31(4):202–7.

3. Singh D, Ferrero A, Rose B, et al. Bone marrow edema syndrome of the foot and ankle: mid- to long-term follow-up in 18 patients. Foot Ankle Spec 2016;9(3):218–26.

4. Curtiss PH Jr, Kincaid WE. Transitory demineralization of the hip in pregnancy. A report of three cases. J Bone Joint Surg Am 1959;41A(7):1327–33.

5. Röhner E, Zippelius T, Steindl D, et al. Effects of intravenous iloprost therapy in patients with bone marrow oedema of the foot and ankle. Eur J Orthop Surg Traumatol 2014;24(8):1609–16.

6. Sprinchorn AE, O'Sullivan R, Beischer AD. Transient bone marrow edema of the foot and ankle and its association with reduced systemic bone mineral density. Foot Ankle Int 2011;32(5):508–12.

7. Bartl C, Imhoff A, Bartl R. Treatment of bone marrow edema syndrome with intravenous ibandronate. Arch Orthop Trauma Surg 2012;132(12):1781–8.

8. Trepman E, King TV. Transient osteoporosis of the hip misdiagnosed as osteonecrosis on magnetic resonance imaging. Orthop Rev 1992;21(9):1089–91, 1094–8.

9. Hungerford MW, Koo KH. Distinguishing bone marrow edema syndrome from osteonecrosis. In: Koo KH, Mont MA, Jones LC, editors. Osteonecrosis. Berlin: Springer-Verlag; 2014. p. 235–8.

10. Finals RC, Jobbe JM. Type-IV hyperlipoproteinaemia and transient osteoporosis. Lancet 1972;2(7783):929.

11. Rozenbaum M, Zinman C, Nagler A, et al. Transient osteoporosis of hip joint with liver cirrhosis. J Rheumatol 1984;11(2):241–3.

12. Tannenbaum H, Esdaile J, Rosenthall L. Joint imaging in regional migratory osteoporosis. J Rheumatol 1979;7(2):237–44.

13. Radke S, Vispo-Seara J, Walther M, et al. Transient bone marrow oedema of the foot. Int Orthop 2001;25(4):263–7.

14. Starr AM, Wessely MA, Albastaki U, et al. Bone marrow edema: pathophysiology, differential diagnosis, and imaging. Acta Radiol 2008;49(7):771–86.

15. Aigner N, Petje G, Steinboeck G, et al. Treatment of bone-marrow oedema of the talus with the prostacyclin analogue iloprost. An MRI-controlled investigation of a new method. J Bone Joint Surg Br 2001;83(6):855–8.

16. Aigner N, Meizer R, Meraner D, et al. Bone marrow edema syndrome in postpartal women: treatment with iloprost. Orthop Clin North Am 2009;40(2):241–7.

17. Berger CE, Kröner AH, Kristen KH, et al. Transient bone marrow edema syndrome of the knee: clinical

and magnetic resonance imaging results at 5 years after core decompression. Arthroscopy 2006;22(8): 866–71.

18. Berger CE, Kröner AH, Minai-Pour MB, et al. Biochemical markers of bone metabolism in bone marrow edema syndrome of the hip. Bone 2003; 33(3):346–51.

19. Hofmann S, Kramer J, Vakil-Adli A, et al. Painful bone marrow edema of the knee: differential diagnosis and therapeutic concepts. Orthop Clin North Am 2004;35(3):321–33.

20. Korompilias AV, Karantanas AH, Lykissas MG, et al. Bone marrow edema syndrome. Skeletal Radiol 2009;38(5):425–36.

21. Limaye R, Tripathy SK, Pathare S, et al. Idiopathic transient osteoporosis of the talus: a cause for unexplained foot and ankle pain. J Foot Ankle Surg 2012;51(5):632–5.

22. Mayerhoefer ME, Kramer J, Breitenseher MJ, et al. Short-term outcome of painful bone marrow oedema of the knee following oral treatment with iloprost or tramadol: results of an exploratory phase II study of 41 patients. Rheumatology (Oxford) 2007;46(9):1460–5.

23. Lakhanpal S, Ginsburg WW, Luthra HS, et al. Transient regional osteoporosis. A study of 56 cases and review of the literature. Ann Intern Med 1987; 106(3):444–50.

24. Boos S, Sigmund G, Huhle P, et al. Magnetic resonance tomography of so-called transient osteoporosis. Primary diagnosis and follow-up after treatment. Rofo 1993;158(3):201–6 [in German].

25. Laroche M, Jacquemier JM, Montane de la Roque P, et al. Nifedipine per os relieves the pain caused by osteonecrosis of the femur head. Rev Rhum Mal Osteoartic 1990;57(9):669–70 [in French].

26. Fernandez-Canton G, Casado O, Capelastegui A, et al. Bone marrow edema syndrome of the foot: one year follow-up with MR imaging. Skeletal Radiol 2003;32(5):273–8.

27. Simon MJ, Barvencik F, Luttke M, et al. Intravenous bisphosphonates and vitamin D in the treatment of bone marrow oedema in professional athletes. Injury 2014;45(6):981–7.

28. Aigner N, Meizer R, Stolz G, et al. Iloprost for the treatment of bone marrow edema in the hindfoot. Foot Ankle Clin 2003;8(4):683–93.

29. Baier C, Schaumburger J, Götz J, et al. Bisphosphonates or prostacyclin in the treatment of bone-marrow oedema syndrome of the knee and foot. Rheumatol Int 2013;33(6):1397–402.

30. Jäger M, Tillmann FP, Thornhill TS, et al. Rationale for prostaglandin I2 in bone marrow oedema: from theory to application. Arthritis Res Ther 2008;10(5): R120.

31. Arazi M, Kiresi D. Bone marrow edema syndrome of the third metatarsal bone: a rare cause of

metatarsalgia treated with iloprost. Eur J Orthop Surg Traumatol 2011;21(1):59–62.

32. Jäger M, Zilkens C, Bittersohl B, et al. Efficiency of iloprost treatment for osseous malperfusion. Int Orthop 2011;35(5):761–5.

33. Ringe JD, Dorst A, Faber H. Effective and rapid treatment of painful localized transient osteoporosis (bone marrow edema) with intravenous ibandronate. Osteoporos Int 2005;16(12):2063–8.

34. Mirghasemi SA, Trepman E, Sadeghi MS, et al. Bone marrow edema syndrome in the foot and ankle. Foot Ankle Int 2016;37(12):1364–73.

35. Rolvien T, Schmidt T, Butscheidt S, et al. Denosumab is effective in the treatment of bone marrow oedema syndrome. Injury 2017;48(4):874–9.

36. Flores-Robles BJ, Sanz-Sanz J, Sanabria-Sanchinel AA, et al. Zoledronic acid treatment in primary bone marrow edema syndrome. J Pain Palliat Care Pharmacother 2017;31(1):52–6.

37. Horas K, Fraissler L, Maier G, et al. High prevalence of vitamin D deficiency in patients with bone marrow edema syndrome of the foot and ankle. Foot Ankle Int 2017;38(7):760–6.

38. Kang S, Gao F, Han J, et al. Extracorporeal shock wave treatment can normalize painful bone marrow edema in knee osteoarthritis: a comparative historical cohort study. Medicine 2018;97(5):e9796.

39. Martinelli N, Bianchi A, Sartorelli E, et al. Treatment of bone marrow edema of the talus with pulsed electromagnetic fields: outcomes in six patients. J Am Podiatr Med Assoc 2015;105(1): 27–32.

40. Ghosh P, inventor; Paradigm Health Sciences Pty Ltd, assignee. Treatment of bone marrow edema (oedema) with polysulfated polysaccharides. Fairlight (AU): United States patent Appl US 15/720,884. 2018.

41. Aigner N, Petje G, Schneider W, et al. Bone marrow edema syndrome of the femoral head: treatment with the prostacyclin analogue iloprost vs. core decompression: an MRI-controlled study. Wien Klin Wochenschr 2005;117(4):130–5.

42. Calvo E, Alvarez L, Fernandez-Yruegas D, et al. Transient osteoporosis of the foot. Bone marrow edema in 4 cases studied with MRI. Acta Orthop Scand 1997;68(6):577–80.

43. Miller JR, Dunn KW. Subchondroplasty of the ankle: a novel technique. Foot Ankle Online J 2015;8(1): 1–7.

44. Kon E, Ronga M, Filardo G, et al. Bone marrow lesions and subchondral bone pathology of the knee. Knee Surg Sports Traumatol Arthrosc 2016;24(6): 1797–814.

45. Bernhard K, Ng A, Kruse D, et al. Surgical treatment of bone marrow lesion associated with recurrent plantar fasciitis: a case report describing an innovative technique using subchondroplasty®. J Foot Ankle Surg 2018;57(4):811–5.

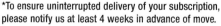

Printed and bound by CPI Group (UK) Ltd, Croydon, CR0 4YY

08/05/2025

01864744-0001

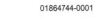